Chiropractic in America

Chiropractic

in America

*The History of
a Medical Alternative*

J. Stuart Moore

The Johns Hopkins University Press

BALTIMORE AND LONDON

© 1993 The Johns Hopkins University Press
All rights reserved
Printed in the United States of America on acid-free paper

The Johns Hopkins University Press
2715 North Charles Street
Baltimore, Maryland 21218-4319
The Johns Hopkins Press Ltd., London

Library of Congress Cataloging-in-Publication Data

Moore, J. Stuart.
   Chiropractic in America : the history of a medical alternative /
J. Stuart Moore.
      p. cm.
   Includes bibliographical references and index.
   ISBN 0-8018-4539-4 (hc : alk. paper)
    1. Chiropractic—United States—History. I. Title.
   [DNLM: 1. Chiropractic—history—United States. WB 905.6M822c]
   RZ225.U6M66 1993
   615.5'34'0973—dc20
   DNLM/DLC
   for Library of Congress   92-48232

A catalog record for this book is available from the British Library.

For Sue, Jeremy, Megan, Mom, and Dad

Contents

Illustrations

Preface

Chiropractors frequently sport license plates that announce SPINEDOC or BACK DR., mobile testimony to the persistence of back pain and related spinal problems in modern-day America. The phrase "oh, my aching back," which has passed into the language as a common expression of exasperation, testifies to the longstanding nature of the problem. American backs *are* aching and have always ached, even though the modes of travel, methods of play, and conditions of labor have all changed dramatically through the years. Nineteenth-century Americans who traveled the rails were subject to a condition known as "railway spine,"[1] a counterpart to twentieth-century automobile whiplash. Although nineteenth-century rural Americans were conditioned by the rigors of farm life, their constant physical exertion created daily opportunities for back injury; even the best conditioning offers little protection against improper lifting or a sudden wrong twist. Farm mechanization at the end of the century may have reduced overt physical strain, but also meant hours spent bouncing on a tractor seat, a jackhammer motion calculated to test the limits of spinal endurance. The sedentary white-collar workplace of the twentieth century, representing a technological liberation from hard labor, helped turn the lifting American of previous generations into the sitting American, a posture that puts almost 50 percent more stress on the spine than standing erect.[2] Weekend athletic feats of present-day, backyard All-Americans who spend their workdays hunched over desks ensure a continual rash of back troubles. The sitting, as well as the lifting and playing American, whether on the farm or in the office, has always been subject to back pain.

According to current estimates, 80 percent of the population will suffer with low back ailments at some point during adult life; on any given day, six million Americans lie in bed wracked with back pain. By the late 1980s, some ninety-three million workdays were lost each year because of back troubles, second only to respiratory infections as a cause of absenteeism. The federal government has estimated the annual bill for treatment and compensation to be fourteen billion dollars, an underestimate according to some health professionals.[3]

Chiropractors play a major role in easing these aching backs and have become the second largest healing group in America (after medical doctors). Unlike the other nonorthodox medical movements of the nineteenth century, chiropractic has not only survived intact, but also flourished. Chiropractic has avoided the oblivion or absorption suffered by other alternative movements. How this happened is the central question of this study.

Because of the current orientation toward back ailments, it would be logical to assume that chiropractic originated as a back specialty in much the same way that dentists emerged as experts for teeth. Logical perhaps, but wrong. The chiropractor's current role as SPINEDOC is an evolved position, a far more restricted role than that envisioned by D.D. Palmer, the founder of chiropractic. He had much more in mind.

Acknowledgments

Scholarly efforts are never solo affairs. I would like to give special thanks to Joseph F. Kett for shepherding this project through its dissertation phase and for helping me to understand that a dissertation need not be plagued with dissertationese. His perceptive advice, insight, and encouragement along the way made this study better than it would have been otherwise. "Keep it up," he wrote after critiquing an early chapter, "and you'll get a book out of this." Aware that he never wrote such things frivolously, I knew at least that I had the wheels on the track. Dorothy Ross, H.C. Erik Midelfort, and Franklyn N. Arnhoff helped to keep them on the track by giving careful attention to the manuscript. Edward Jervey, my now-retired (but not retiring) colleague at Radford University, also read the manuscript with his characteristic gusto and continues to be a source of support.

Librarians and archivists are crucial to such endeavors and deserve a special dispensation of grace. I regret that I do not know the names of all those who helped me (especially those at the National Library of Medicine at Bethesda, Maryland), but special thanks to Glenda Wiese, Archivist at the Daniel David Palmer Health Sciences Library, Palmer College of Chiropractic, Davenport, Iowa; Rosemary Buhr, Director, Learning Resources Center, and Arthur L. (now deceased) and Vi Nixon, Archivists (and gracious hosts), Logan College of Chiropractic, Chesterfield, Missouri; Ann MacGregor, Health Sciences Library, College of Health Sciences, Roanoke, Virginia; and Clayne Calhoun, Roanoke Law Library, Roanoke, Virginia.

A special thanks to William Rehm, D.C., who was always willing to loan me whatever materials I requested from his own personal holdings and from the archives of the Association for the History of Chiropractic. Special thanks also to George P. McAndrews, principal attorney for the plaintiffs in the Wilk case, for supplying me with a packet of materials that was especially helpful. While in the research phase, my in-laws, Price and Marie Ransone of Towson, Maryland, were happy to house and feed my family during my trips to Bethesda. Such hospitality and good cheer are crucial for anyone engaged in research.

The editor at Johns Hopkins Press, Jacqueline Wehmueller, and the manuscript editor, Linda Forlifer, made the process of turning a pile of manuscript pages into a book as painless as possible and handled the project with diligence and care. Thank you.

I owe a great debt to my parents, Clarence and Sarah Moore, who have always supported and nurtured me. I owe one equally as great to my wife Sue, who always believed in and encouraged me and somehow managed to get a master's degree and work full time while I was in the midst of this. And finally to Jeremy and Megan, a hope that one day you'll be able to really understand what Daddy has been up to for the past seven years. Until then, any mistakes that remain in this work are their fault.

Chiropractic in America

Chapter One

Subluxations, Science, and the Spine: D.D. Palmer and the Origins of Chiropractic

Science is knowledge; ascertained facts; accumulated information of causes and principles systematized. I ascertained these truths, acquired instruction, heretofore unrecognized, regarding the performance of functions in health and disease. I systematized and correlated these principles, made them practical. By doing so I created, brought into existence, originated a science, which I named Chiropractic; therefore I am a scientist. I systematized the principles I discovered; I have reasoned from cause to effect; searched into the nature of physiologic and pathologic processes; investigated the phenomena embraced in health and disease; assigned rational causes for the existence of normal and abnormal functions; answered the question, "What is life"; and founded a science and philosophy upon the basic principle of tone. This knowledge I have given to the world; therefore I am a philosopher.
    D.D. Palmer, *The Science, Art and Philosophy of Chiropractic*

Medicine says, all is matter, never mind.
Christian Science says, There's mind, never matter.
But Chiropractic says, There's mind, working through matter.
                    Unattributed chiropractic aphorism

THE FIRST ADJUSTMENT

"Cures without Medicine" proclaimed an advertisement for D.D. Palmer in the 1887 Davenport, Iowa, City Directory.[1] In his quest for the cause and cure of disease, Daniel David Palmer, self-anointed spiritualist and magnetic healer, had embraced a drugless approach to health which would lead him to devise a novel alternative to regular medicine. "One question was uppermost in my mind in my search for the cause of disease," Palmer wrote. "I desired to know why one person was ailing, and his associate, eating at the same table, working in the same shop, at the same bench, was not. Why? . . . This question had worried thousands for centuries and was answered in September, 1895."[2] Palmer gave his first spinal adjustment to Harvey Lillard, a deaf black janitor for the Ryan Building in Davenport, where Palmer retained an office. "The First Adjustment," on September 18, has assumed mythic proportions in chiropractic lore, best illustrated by the masthead on B.J. Palmer's periodical publication, *Fountain Head News,* which dates time itself from 1895. For example, 1910 becomes "15 A.C." (fifteenth year "After Chiropractic").

By the time Palmer penned his most elaborate description of the incident in his erratic 1910 tome *The Science, Art and Philosophy of Chiropractic* or *The Chiropractor's Adjuster,* several earlier accounts and circulating rumors had described the Lillard adjustment as an accidental discovery, the result of a lucky happenstance.[3] Palmer became defensive in attempting to dispel these notions and insisted on the scientific nature of his manipulation. According to Palmer, Lillard

> had been so deaf for 17 years that he could not hear the racket of a wagon or the ticking of a watch. I made inquiry as to the cause of his deafness and was informed that when he was exerting himself in a cramped, stooped position, he felt something give way in his back and immediately became deaf. An examination showed a vertebra racked from its normal position. I reasoned that if that vertebra was replaced, the man's hearing should be restored. With this object in view, a half-hour's talk persuaded Mr. Lillard to allow me to replace it. I racked it into position by using the spinous process as a lever and soon the man could hear as before. There was nothing "accidental" about this, as it was accomplished with an object in view, and the expected was obtained. There was nothing "crude" about this adjustment; it was specific, so much so that no Chiropractor has equaled it.[4]

Although Palmer's account probably condenses what were actually a series of manipulative attempts on Lillard, his scientific posture undoubtedly came from a desire to escape his reputation as a quack practitioner and to associate himself with the rising fortunes of science.[5] On May 13, 1894, the *Davenport Leader,* in a piece entitled simply "Dr. Palmer," had dismissed him as a charlatan who preyed on simpletons.

> A crank on magnetism, [Palmer] has a crazy notion that he can cure the sick and crippled by his magnetic hands. His victims are the weak-minded, ignorant and superstitious, those foolish people who have been sick for years

and have become tired of the regular physician and want health by a short-cut method. . . . He exerts a wonderful magnetic power over his patients, making many of them believe they are well. His increase in business shows what can be done in Davenport even by a quack.[6]

Such charges of quackery were nothing new. In a case attracting wide local publicity and affording considerable amusement to courtroom spectators in November 1890, Palmer sued one Nicholas Wiltamuth of Moline, Illinois, for partial nonpayment of a magnetic healing bill. The defense charged that Palmer was a quack without a diploma from a medical college or a license to practice. Palmer stressed his contractual arrangement with the defendant, claimed that his practice was not the practice of medicine, and, according to the *Moline Dispatch* account of November 15, 1890, noted that he held a diploma "from no earthly school but from High Heaven." "Considerable curiosity was manifested as to the diploma," continued the *Dispatch,* "but it was not produced for inspection." Palmer eventually won the case in a subsequent trial and was awarded $20, the balance of the original, unpaid bill. Nonetheless, his reputation as a mountebank persisted.[7]

No one enjoys the quack label, and Palmer was determined that his new brainchild, chiropractic, would acquire the scientific respectability that his earlier career in spiritualism and magnetic healing had lacked. For one with spiritual leanings untempered by formal scientific training, it was a Herculean task.

The Early Days of D.D. Palmer

"When a baby," D.D. Palmer wrote, tapping the best frontier tradition of the Canadian west, "I was cradled in a piece of hemlock bark." He was born on March 7, 1845, a few miles northeast of Toronto in a quaint hamlet on the shore of Lake Scugog, later known as Port Perry. At the time, Palmer noted, it was "away out west."[8]

A mother who was "as full of superstition as an egg is full of meat" nurtured his sensitive nature while a father who was "disposed to reason on the subjects pertaining to life" schooled him in the practical art of rational thinking.[9] His formal instruction by a country schoolmaster was interrupted in 1856 when his father's business failure forced a family move to the United States. However, D.D. and his younger brother Thomas were left behind to work in a stave and match factory, and schooling became intermittent. Not until April 1865 did the brothers set out for the United States with two borrowed dollars. Traveling through Buffalo, Detroit, and Chicago, they rejoined their family 2½ months later in Iowa.[10]

Eight months after his arrival, D.D. began teaching in Muscatine, a career that led him to assignments in several Iowa counties and in 1871 to a community school in New Boston, Illinois. In his journal, D.D. carefully recorded the names of his pupils and their ages (ranging from five to twenty-one) and a list of aphorisms for teaching which illustrate some of his difficulties. These include "Simplify all subjects for the young," "Whip giving time between the strokes," "Use persuasion to get large boys to quit using tobacco," "The quietest schools study the most," and the time-honored admonition, "Tell pupils to not look cross for looks will stay." Also in the journal is a page entitled "Mottoes," which indicate his approach to life. Included are "Study first, play afterwards, Truth always"; "Study hours. Find a way or make a way"; "Use a book as a bee does a flower"; and "The best physicians are Dr. Diet, Dr. Quiet, and Dr. Merryman."[11]

After purchasing ten hillside acres north of New Boston, Palmer began a new venture as horticulturist and apiarist. A stickler for detail, he kept extensive notes on his planting and beekeeping activities. For a decade his carefully cultivated "Sweet Home raspberry" found a nationwide market, while his bees in some years produced several thousand pounds of honey. A harsh winter in 1881, with temperatures dipping to twenty and thirty below zero, ended the apiary. Concise and detached, Palmer recorded the event in his journal: "Bees all dead."

Apparently disheartened, Palmer sold his New Boston property in December 1881 and rejoined his parents, brothers, and sisters at What Cheer, Iowa, a booming coal town seventy-five miles west of the Mississippi. Palmer opened a grocery store offering goldfish as well as more traditional wares, but competition pushed him back into itinerant teaching. Restless and unsettled, he moved to Letts, Iowa, and began searching for a career more suited to his temperament and more conducive to a steady income.

SPIRITUALISM, MAGNETIC HEALING, AND THE HARMONIAL TRADITION

D.D. Palmer had been fascinated by spiritualism for many years. Popularized by Kate and Margaret Fox in the 1840s, the possibility of communing with the dead drew attention from both serious investigators and psychic dilettantes in parlors across the nation.[12] While in New Boston, Palmer cultivated an avid interest in the new religious movement and even incorporated his spiritual views on the front and inside cover of a forty-page nursery catalog. In addition to advertising his various raspberry varieties, Palmer clearly identified himself as a spiritualist who sought to expose the psychic tomfoolery at Mott's, a spiritualist resort in Memphis, Missouri, which "preys upon the purse of the honest investigator and makes a mockery of that to all most dear, the future existence of those who have passed from earth life."[13] Palmer was assuming the role of an authentic spiritualist and to him such charlatanry threatened to discredit legitimate spiritual phenomena.

What actually confronted D.D. Palmer as he began his career search in earnest was the problem of assimilating spirit to science while avoiding the spurious, "unscientific" spiritualist mire. By eventually traveling a path from spiritualism through magnetic healing to his innovation of chiropractic, Palmer tapped into the harmonial tradition (which in America dates at least from Emerson), an impulse with certain affinities to the centuries-old hermetic tradition.[14] Palmer's ideas stood clearly within the harmonial tradition, an association that would serve to buttress his often erratic thought and idiosyncratic expression.

Determining the lineage and boundaries of traditions is a precarious task. "We cannot understand theories if we confine them in a temporal straightjacket," medical historian Lester King noted. "Theories have deep roots, lost in antiquity, and nowhere is this more true than in medicine."[15] As early as the fifth century B.C., Plato, who emphasized the preeminence of the immaterial world, and Democritus, who championed the material world as primary reality, drew the battle lines that ever since have animated arguments in Western medical theory over the relationship between *spiritus* and *materia*.[16] The fundamental premise of harmonial thought in America, the immediate backdrop for Palmer's notions, is the coinherence of Matter and Spirit. Harmonialism can be defined as a form of piety in which believers understand themselves as part of a great Cosmic Ocean, that All are really subsumed in One. Getting "in tune with the Infinite" becomes the central, critical task for adherents. Cosmic rapport ensures not only spiritual well-being but also physical health and even economic success. In 1897, Ralph Waldo Trine provided a classic explanation of harmonial thought.

> There is a divine sequence running throughout the universe. Within and above and below the human will incessantly works the Divine will. To come into harmony with it and thereby with all the higher laws and forces, to come then into league and to work in conjunction with them, in order that they can work in league and conjunction with us, is to come into the chain of this wonderful sequence. This is the secret of all success. This is to come into possession of unknown riches, into the realization of undreamed-of powers.[17]

Historian Robert Fuller distinguished two main temperaments within the harmonial tradition of American Protestantism—the "ascetic," who yearned for cosmic harmony but was tempered by orthodox religious thinking and Biblical piety, and the "aesthetic," who longed for a "progressive, co-scientific religious outlook" unrestrained by traditional Christian morality.[18] Both of these types would eventually find their way into the chiropractic fold and create controversy over the relationship of chiropractic to Christianity.

Palmer himself took the aesthetic approach. His version of harmonial piety took root in his spiritualist dabblings, an excursion that prepared him for the tenets of magnetic healing, a harmonial-style therapy that sought to channel divine curative forces. Although unknown to Palmer, Paracelsus (1493–1541), astrologer and physician, stands as an important precursor for those who would later seek to direct metaphysical energy for healing. In Paracelsus's age, the traditional view (inherited from Galen) that health resulted from a proper balance of the four "cardinal humors" (blood, phlegm, choler, and melancholy) still informed medical understanding. According to this time-honored view, either an excess or a deficiency of one or more humors meant disease. In contrast, Paracelsus taught that disease came from specific causes outside of the body and that the body itself was not a battleground for the humors, but rather a harmonious microcosm animated by a vital force that he termed the *Archeus*. All matter, both organic and inorganic, had its own Archeus, which worked to expel harmful substances (primarily poisons flowing from stars in the atmosphere) and thus preserve and enhance life. This natural force, however, could be stymied by inharmonious thought and action. It was the task of the physician, "a god of the Little World [of men], appointed as God's deputy" to help the Archeus cast out the poisonous intruders, with specific medicines or with words. God, by the force of nature, cured.[19]

Paracelsus also taught that a type of magnetic aura emanated from humans, capable of attracting both good and evil, and by an act of the will could be used to influence others. Joan Baptista Van Helmont (1579–1644), a physician and alchemist who intended to demolish the traditional Galenic system, advanced this concept by adding the idea that a specific life-force, an indigenous *archeus insitus*, existed for each major organ of the body.[20] Numerous healers soon invoked "animal magnetism" (from the Latin *anima*, meaning soul) to aid in effecting cures. Scottish doctor William Maxwell endorsed the magnetic ideas of Van Helmont in *De medicina magnetica* (published in 1679 but written years earlier),[21] while Englishman Robert Fludd (1574–1637), a "philosophical physician," helped to battle the emerging mechanical philosophy of nature.[22]

In the context of the late Renaissance and the early seventeenth century, this vitalistic approach to the world was rooted in the science of its day. Astrology, for example, was in part an intricate mathematical science based on the idea that the position of the stars at the time of birth disclosed a preordained future. Magic became a way of escaping from astral determinism by directing the influences of the stars in desired directions and was, in a religious sense, a way of salvation.[23]

Gabriel Naudé, a celebrated man of letters and bibliographer, distinguished four kinds of magic in his famous *Apology for Great Men Suspected of Magic* (1625). Divine magic was beyond human manipulation, theurgic or religious magic could liberate the soul from bodily corruption, natural magic was a science based on nature, and goetia was black magic or witchcraft and the only illicit type of the four. According to Naudé, Aristotle and other Greeks had actually practiced natural magic but never mentioned the term magic.[24] Historian Herbert Butterfield warned that: "little progress can be made if we think of the older studies as merely a case of bad science or if we imagine that only the achievements of the scientist in very recent times are worthy of serious attention at the present day."[25] For one imbued with the instincts of vitalism, no real separation between physics and metaphysics existed. An investigator who confined himself to the visible world without reference to the invisible was considered a mere superficial, mechanical tinkerer.

At the dawn of the scientific revolution, the vitalistic approach, which sought to reveal the interpenetration of Spirit and Nature, competed with an emerging mechanical view, which focused on the visible world of Nature. The older tradition became submerged in the undercurrents of the mechanistic "new science" but remained an important legacy that could resurface.

Animal magnetism reemerged, now on the outskirts of science, in the work of Austrian physician Friedrich Anton Mesmer (1734–1815), ushering in the age of mesmerism. Of the numerous systems of the world, mesmerism was most closely aligned with the many vitalistic theories since Paracelsus. Mesmer's opponents clearly recognized him as a scientific descendant of Paracelsus, J.B. Van Helmont, William Maxwell, and Robert Fludd, as one who also tapped the harmonial tradition of correspondence between the microcosm of the individual and the celestial macrocosm. Mesmer believed that he had discovered an invisible fluid, an "agent of nature" that penetrated and encircled all bodies in the universe and was the medium, for example, through which gravity operated on celestial bodies. The human body had "poles" that acted as a type of magnet; an "obstacle" that interrupted the flow of the fluid through the human body meant sickness. Through "mesmerizing" or massaging the body's poles, the operator could overcome the obstacle by directing the action of the fluid and inducing a "crisis" (frequently convulsions) resulting in health, the harmonious restoration of human being and nature.[26] The vigorously named Austrian Committee to Sustain Morality investigated Mesmer's techniques and charged him with creating doctor-patient relationships that led to immoral conduct. Forced from Vienna, Mesmer fled to Switzerland and then to Paris in 1778.[27]

In prerevolutionary France, science was the passionate topic and mesmerism created a major sensation. It offered a serious explanation of Nature to the French, even suggesting wider applications to the forces directing society and politics. Mesmerism was no irrational fancy. Science had only recently revealed a host of miraculous, invisible forces such as Newton's gravity, Franklin's electricity, and astonishing gases that had lifted Pilâtre de Rozier, the first "aeronaute," high over Metz in a balloon in October 1783, the first human flight. Mesmer's fluid was no more wondrous than these. Mesmerism flowed from the recent scientific discoveries and held the promise of a modern spiritualist science, a "haute science" or high science, which could explain root causes. In its beginning phase, it expressed an extreme form of the Enlightenment faith in reason. Yet a confusion of terms among enthusiasts sometimes clouded the ultimate goals of mesmerism. One contemporary mesmerist explained that "physics would take the place of magic everywhere"; another argued that "above science is magic, because magic follows it, not as an effect, but as its perfection." It was the problem of discerning the relationship between physics and metaphysics, Nature and Spirit. Even the most occult followers, however, placed themselves in the scientific stream of the century.[28]

Interest in animal magnetism continued in France despite several official failures (including a Parisian commission initiated by Louis XVI in 1784 and headed by Benjamin Franklin) to discover any therapeutic or scientific validity in Mesmer's approach. By the late 1780s, an eclectic, spiritualist brand of mesmerism began to dominate the movement. "Fluidists" such as Mesmer himself, who believed in an actual, material fluid as a transmitting agent of Nature, were tagged as old-fashioned by the spiritualist wing, who warned that emphasizing the fluid could lead to materialism. Mesmer had lost control of his movement; it was moving throughout Europe into supernatural realms that he had sought to avoid. A revival of mesmerism in the mid–nineteenth century tilted heavily toward spiritualism.[29]

John Elliotson (1791–1868), the renowned English physician and professor of medicine at University College, London, lent his considerable prestige to the movement and hoped to give respectability to mesmeric concepts by culling effective therapeutic uses. In 1843 he inaugurated the journal *Zoist* and attempted, in effect, to rescue mesmerism from its spiritualist components. The spiritualist implications, however, were too compelling to avoid, and Elliotson and his fellow contributors often lapsed into abstractions concerning ultimate causes. Elliotson found anesthetic surgical uses for mesmerism and detailed his successes in *Numerous Cases of Surgical Operations without Pain in the Mesmeric State,* an 1843 polemic published in Philadelphia, but the discovery of ether provided a more respectable method for relieving pain. *Zoist,* the only outlet for reports of mesmeric therapy, folded in 1856, leaving mesmerism and magnetic healing no place to go except down the road to spiritualism.[30]

But the tenets of magnetic healing survived, in a pared-down mix of Spirit and Matter which became especially popular in America. Frenchman Charles Poyen had introduced mesmerism to the American public in the mid-1830s by traveling the lecture circuit in the Northeast. An August 1836 address by Poyen in Bangor, Maine, roused listener Phineas Parkhurst Quimby, who subsequently established a longstanding healing practice. In 1862 Quimby treated Mary Baker Eddy,[31] the founder of Christian Science, who spun the spiritualist aspect of mesmerism to its logical, extreme conclusion—denial of the existence of Matter. It was possible, of course, to embrace the power of magnetic healing without completely disowning Matter. By retaining a material component reminiscent of Mesmer's position, a magnetic operator could lay claim to the title of high scientist in its historic sense, as one who understood the movement of *spiritus* within *materia*. By the late nineteenth century, however, this conjunction of Spirit and Matter was increasingly anachronistic as science distanced itself from metaphysics. Elliotson, the respected scientist, had failed in his attempt to recapture the ground lost to the spiritualist camp, and the rescue descended to a more popular level, where results and techniques were often more important than theory. D.D. Palmer, marching under the banner of science, immersed himself in a popularized version of magnetic healing which invoked these sometimes vague, material powers of the universe and learned to direct them with proper technique—a type of poor man's mesmerism.[32]

Palmer was impressed by the stature of a magnetic healer named Paul Caster, who worked out of Ottumwa, Iowa, in the 1870s and was known locally as a faith doctor. Caster's large practice netted a tidy fortune; according to his 1881 obituary his "fame brought invalids from every corner of the earth almost. . . . In one of his rooms to-day you will find a wagon load of crutches, canes and other kindred devices, left as mute witness of his success in an inexplicable practice. . . . He was always recognized as an honest man, and had he been blessed with an education, there is no telling what hight [*sic*] his eminence might have reached."[33] Caster's son J.S., a machinist for the Chicago, Burlington & Quincy Railroad, eventually assumed the magnetic trade in the Mississippi River town of Burlington, Iowa, and like his father drew thousands of patients and public acclaim in an area that was fast becoming a magnetic Mecca. The restless D.D. Palmer saw his opportunity. He moved to Burlington, and in September 1886 opened a magnetic healing business in three rooms at 408 ½ Jefferson Street. Competition from assorted eclectics, homeopaths, botanics, and occultists, however, pushed Palmer to seek another locality. By

1887, Palmer had shifted his fledgling practice to Davenport, seventy-five miles upriver, and began his drugless cures in earnest. His move may also have been prompted by an unhappy family situation and the demands of a large ego. His daybook (September 3, 1886 through August 12, 1887) includes a note dated October 13, 1886, next to the name "Bart," probably his brother and presumably from him. It reads: "Three rules to be observed that success may attend you. 1st Be not deceived by women, 3 times have they been a curse morally, physically and financially. 2nd The less you talk the more you will accomplish and the greater importance will be attached to your cures. 3rd Remember you did not come here for your health or glory alone, it will not feed you or your children."[34]

How Palmer attempted to cure is revealed by the books and manuals he possessed which instructed aspiring healers on proper magnetic principles and techniques. C.A. DeGroodt of Burlington, in his *Hygeio-Therapeutic Institute and Magnetic Infirmary*, wrote effusively of "the grandest, the most subtile and refined force operating in human affairs—the vital Aura, the direct interpreter of life itself—the force called MAGNETISM; a principle so subtile that it can search through and through all other substances, and even use electricity itself in its mission among men." Degroodt described himself as a "magnetic physician," one who used the biblical gift of healing by directing scientific forces. He was no mere faith healer performing miracles, but a scientist using a spiritual gift that could bend the sternest will. "Do not think because you have no faith in my way of doctoring that I will not cure you," Degroodt explained smugly, "for when you are once cured, you must have faith in my way of doctoring."[35]

Palmer learned rules for treatment from his copy of *Vital Magnetism, The Life Fountain* (n.d., c. mid-1870s), a handbook for the magnetist by E.D. Babbitt, D.M. (apparently Doctor of Magnetism).

1. Make passes from *heated* or *inflamed parts,* toward the extremities or cold parts.
2. Give a new tide of life to *cold negative parts,* by holding, rubbing, or spatting them.
3. Place the *right hand,* which is positive, on the hot part, and the *left,* or *negative hand,* on the cool, on the principle that forces flow from positive to negative. Reverse this order in thoroughly left-handed persons.
4. If the system is *dormant,* as in *Chronic Rheumatism, Paralysis,* etc., *upward* movements are very important as assisting the *capillary* action. Pass up all the limbs and spine, but avoid upward passes near the head. Vitalize the back-neck, and shoulders thoroughly, make passes from the hips upward diagonally to the shoulders, and animate the portions back and front of the ears thoroughly.

Babbitt continued with instructions on the proper passes for liver, stomach, lung, heart, and kidney ailments, as well as techniques for relieving costiveness (constipation), diarrhea, headache, convulsions, apoplexy, and sunstroke. "To quicken a dull intellect" Babbitt advised the magnetic operator to "rub the forehead, brows, and temples." Rubbing the top and front of the head would "animate the moral powers," while passing from the back of the head and neck down the shoulders and arms "would scatter extra heat in the passional region." To cover any ostensible ill-effects of treatment, Babbitt offered an ambiguous warning that could apply to the patient, the magnetist, or both. "When the magnetist arouses a dormant system, do not be alarmed if you feel worse for a while."

In concluding this portion of his manual, Babbitt gave the aspiring healer hints for developing magnetic power. "Cultivate a true and pure life. . . . It is impossible to gain the finest and most penetrating aura and live a base and selfish life. It should be remembered that this vital aura partakes of the nature of both soul and body. A low nature can treat only low people as a general rule." On a practical level this admonition meant receiving treatments from an established magnetist (which served to enhance magnetic force), exercising outdoors, sleeping with the head to the north "to be in harmony with the earth's magnetic and electric currents," eating fruits, vegetables, and cereals rather than meats and spices, avoiding "all debasing stimuli" such as tobacco and liquor, and hand bathing in cool water upon rising and retiring. In a passage marked by Palmer, Babbitt advised sitting quietly every night with closed eyes, "remaining receptive to the great ocean of fine spiritual atmosphere about you, and with silent prayer seek for higher influences." Babbitt warned, however, that such an exercise had its pitfalls. "On pursuing that course my head has become so electrical that I have not dared to place my hand upon it. This is a refining process and may cause some suffering for a while, but it is the pathway to power." It also served as a career guide, a barometer of magnetic potential. "If, after sitting in this way a few days or weeks your head receives no pressure of electricity, you had probably better not attempt to become a professional magnetist, as you would be liable to become exhausted in treating others continuously." In a later passage that must have impressed Palmer, Babbitt noted that "*the small of the back* is an important point for manipulations, sometimes in the circular, but sometimes in horizontal movements."[36]

Palmer owned other works that taught principles and procedures similar to those detailed by DeGroodt and Babbitt. Some had the same practical mentality, such as *How to Magnetize, or Magnetism and Clairvoyance* and *How to Mesmerize, Ancient and Modern Miracles by Mesmerism: Also Is Spiritualism True?* Others had a more academic flavor but retained the how-to approach—*A Lecture on the Philosophy of Disease, and How to Cure the Sick without Drugs, with an Explanation of Magnetic Laws, A Lecture on Life and Health, or How to Live a Century,* and *Psychometry and Thought-*

Transference, with Practical Hints for Experiments, the latter printed in Boston, appropriately by the Esoteric Publishing Company.[37]

One last title merits special mention, the *Fruits of Philosophy: A Treatise on the Population Question*, a noted pamphlet on contraceptive technique published originally in 1832 by Boston physician Charles Knowlton but suppressed in the United States. The edition Palmer owned was published by Charles Bradlaugh and Theosophist Anne Besant specifically to test the right of publication, and its distribution occasioned a trial in 1877. It is quite possible that Palmer's magnetic practice included birth control advice—periodically his daybook shows an entry "adv." in the treatment column. For example, on Sunday, January 24, 1892, he saw "A Belgian Woman" and gave advice. On another occasion "A Woman" paid four dollars (four times the rate for a typical treatment) for fifteen minutes worth of "adv." That he did not enter their names is especially arresting since the vast majority of his patients were entered by name in his daybook.

After poring over his books, Palmer became convinced that he possessed the gift of healing. His lack of formal education was certainly no hindrance in the still laissez-faire medical marketplace of the late nineteenth century, especially in rural America where education beyond the basics continued to be suspect. The laissez-faire medical scene (especially regarding magnetic healing practitioners) is illustrated by the so-called McAnnulty rule, arising at the turn of the century out of a Supreme Court case pitting J.H. Kelly and his American School of Magnetic Healing against the postmaster of Nevada, Missouri (J.M. McAnnulty). In effect, the rule formally sanctioned a laissez-faire marketplace for unorthodox practitioners of all stripes. In siding with Kelly (who claimed to cure by a "practical scientific system" of magnetic mail-order therapy), Justice Rufus W. Peckham ruled that the lack of exact standards of therapeutic efficacy and the multitude of conflicting medical opinions meant that determination of fraud was beyond the purview of the Postmaster General, who had wrongfully withheld delivery of mail to Kelly and his school. The ruling made subsequent charges of fraud extremely difficult to prove with regard to any type of therapy.[38]

Palmer opened the "Magnetic Cure and Infirmary" in the Ryan Building on the corner of Second and Brady Streets in Davenport and with aggressive advertising began to develop a lucrative practice. Because his office was only two blocks from a Mississippi River ferry, he drew his clientele not only from Iowa towns such as Sweetland Center, Blue Grass, White Sulphur, and Newton, but also from places in Illinois such as Yellow Creek, Galva, Geneseo, and Lanark. Palmer treated ailments ranging from "general debility," rheumatism, bad backs, neuralgia, and malaria to indigestion, sore throat, toothache, and worms. Although he gave a number of free treatments, his in-office regimen usually went for one dollar with payment or nonpayment carefully recorded by Palmer in his daybook. Cash receipts jumped from $700 in 1887 to $2,507 in 1890 to $4,669 in 1895, at a time when the average physician's income ranged between $1,000 and $1,500.[39]

Palmer's success convinced him that the drugless approach was therapeutically valid—his patients would not continue to pay if they failed to benefit. His magnetic practice became the training ground for the coming of chiropractic, a practice that had tapped into the vitalistic, spiritualist track essential to Palmer's developing theory of disease. Already in magnetic healing there were glimpses of the importance of the spine, "nerve power," and of the operator's touch in the curative process. But the soul and hand cure of magnetism was topheavy with soul. There was another track leading to chiropractic, which emphasized the purely mechanical act of hand manipulation. This tradition—bonesetting—also had a metaphysical air, but these medical tradesmen usually concentrated on the practical art of replacing dislocations and left cosmic matters to the speculations of others. In any case, Palmer failed to give bonesetting due credit. "Chiropractic," he argued, "was not evolved from medicine or from any other method, except that of magnetic." He remained intent on establishing the novelty of his "discovery": "Chiropractic is a new profession, all others are old and crowded."[40]

"The Wrench and the Rough Movement": Manipulators and Bonesetters

Manual manipulation of the joints has an ancient heritage. Hippocrates (born 460 B.C.), the legendary Father of Medicine who emphasized the healing force of nature, wrote extensively on techniques for reducing dislocated joints, including "On the Articulations" and "Instruments of Reduction." These treatises were practical manuals intended to assist the practitioner in the workaday art of manipulation. They were not for the fainthearted. For example, to correct chronic shoulder dislocations, Hippocrates advised cauterizing the shoulder by passing hot, oblong irons through the skin of the armpit "burnt to the opposite side" and "pushed forward with the hand; the cauteries should be red-hot, that they may pass through as quickly as possible." He also described methods for reducing displacements of the vertebrae and suggested employing a bench for treatment "six cubits long, two cubits broad, one fathom in thickness, having two low axles at this end and that" and in the middle "excavations like trays," which suggest a prototype of a modern chiropractic adjustment table. (Some chiropractors even claim that chiropractic is the rebirth of Hippocratic techniques.) Clearly, manual manipulation was part of the repertoire of the respectable physician.[41]

Asklepiades, prominent Greek physician in Rome (*circa* 100–50 B.C.), included massage of the spinal column as an important part of his therapeutic regimen.[42] In the second century A.D. Galen, the celebrated Greek doctor and philosopher, won the title "Prince of Physicians" by curing a paralysis of the right hand of Roman scholar Eudemus, apparently by adjusting the vertebrae of the neck.[43] Emerging from such a background, the art of manual manipulation became an important option for trained European physicians. Avicenna of Baghdad, interpreter and preserver of classical literature during the Middle Ages, included the Hippocratic manipulative methods in his medical canon, published numerous times in Europe between 1473 and 1608 in Latin translation. Influential physician Ambroise Paré (1510–90) practiced spinal manipulation and repeated the techniques of Hippocrates in his writings on the dislocation of vertebrae. Johann Schultes (Johannis Scultetus) continued the manipulative tradition in the seventeenth century with *The Surgeons Store-House,* published in London in 1674. By the eighteenth century, however, manipulation was being abandoned by the orthodox. The major reasons for this rejection seem to be a growing awareness during this era that force applied to weakened, tubercular joints (a flourishing malady in the dank, crowded cities) could result in horrible maiming, along with a growing fear of physical contact with contagious patients who could transmit virulent social diseases. Academically untrained "bonesetters" such as Sarah "Crazy Sally" Mapp (a notorious early eighteenth-century English bonesetter famous for kneading posteriors) and assorted folk manipulators stepped in and filled the vacuum by catering to a clientele that still demanded such services.[44] Manual manipulation was deserted by the medical establishment, went underground, and became the sole province of folk practitioners.

Bonesetting had a long heritage among the humble. Between 1530 and 1580 seventeen editions of Friar Thomas Moulton's vernacular *The Mirror or Glass of Health* circulated among the lay public; in 1656 this was revised and enlarged by Robert Turner and published in London as *The Compleat Bone-setter.*[45] Although such a text would appear to extend the practice of bonesetting throughout lay medical culture, the influence of the book in disseminating information was probably minimal. Despite the comprehensive treatment suggested by the title, the book devoted most of its pages to topics tangential to bonesetting. An aspiring manipulator hoping to master the trade by poring over *The Compleat Bone-setter* would instead be completely disappointed. Books were probably beyond the intellectual reach of the public, and as in other skilled trades the tradition passed from father to son largely by direct observation and through practice attended by the keen eye of the master.[46] The homespun nature of the book may have contributed to the abandonment of manipulation by orthodox practitioners by suggesting that such practice was beneath their dignity.

The medical establishment came to identify bonesetters with the ignorant peasantry, and they were denounced by many physicians as mere bone mechanics who treated every injured joint as "put-out" and "put in again," always by the same method, "the wrench and the rough movement."[47]

But European physicians offered few alternatives and censured these techniques largely because they found difficulty in adjusting the deformities treated with some success by the bonesetters. American physicians echoed this attitude and, by the time a medical establishment had developed in America, the skill of manipulation had long since passed out of the armamentarium of the orthodox physician. As Dr. J.B. Brown, founder of the first orthopedic hospital in America (Boston Orthopedic, 1837), noted, "Regular surgeons, finding the uncertainty, difficulty, and frequent impossibility, of curing these [orthopedic] deformities, had relinquished the practice of orthopedy to these ignorant men, who applied such means as their cupidity or stupidity might suggest."[48] A respected tradition of manual medicine never really existed in America; manipulation was wholly the field of the quack and the folk practitioner.

The deans of the bonesetting folk in America were the Sweets of New England. Several generations ministered to the ailing in southern Rhode Island, Connecticut, Massachusetts, and New York. The family gained a considerable reputation when Job Sweet (born 1724) successfully manipulated French Army officers in Newport during the Revolution and later set the dislocated hip of Colonel Aaron Burr's beloved daughter, Theodosia.[49] Job's success enabled him to practice virtually full time, but most of the Sweets labored at traditional occupations such as farming or blacksmithing and set bones as a sideline, occasionally taking their services on the road. The *Daily Pittsburgh Gazette* for November 9, 1837, noted that "natural Bonesetter" Waterman Sweet would arrive shortly to commence work.[50]

Although the success of the Sweets was sometimes attributed by observers to a genetic inner vision enabling them to "see" the bones of the body, their expertise came from more mundane, mechanical means. D.D. Palmer, who was aware of the bonesetters and fashioned himself a medical underdog in the same tradition, related the method that "Old Doctor" Sweet of Sag Harbor used to gain his skill.

> On one occasion [Sweet] was asked by a physician where and how he got the knack or talent of setting bones. He replied: "Don't know; just came to me all of a sudden one day when I had caught a chicken and was about to kill it and first thing I knew, I'd pulled a bone out of place. In putting it back I pulled another out of place, and I pulled another out of place in putting that back. Then, when I'd got 'em all back in place, I got an idea I'd learn how to set bones and give up farming. So, I practiced uncoupling and coupling up the bones of my dog until I learned

the right twists for setting all the different bones. Guess I took the dog apart nigh onto a hundred times, on and off. He got so used to it that he seemed to enjoy it, and I do believe he missed the exercise when I let up on him."[51]

The story itself may be apocryphal, but the hands-on practice and repetition described the genesis of the bonesetter's skill, a skill that came from applied experimentation rather than from books, mystic inner visions, or genes. For D.D. Palmer such work was not the undignified tinkering of the ignorant but a practical means of advancing a natural science that was ignored by an ossified medical establishment. "It is a pity that the medical profession are possessed of arrogance instead of liberality," Palmer wrote after a complimentary discussion of the bonesetters, "that instead of encouraging and fostering advanced ideas, they stifle and discourage advancement; that they only adopt advanced ideas when they are compelled to do so by public opinion."[52]

One American medical doctor, Andrew Taylor Still (1828–1917), did abandon orthodox practice for the cause of manual manipulation and established osteopathy, an alternative medical sect that stands as the most important progenitor of chiropractic. Like Palmer, Still had dabbled in magnetic healing and spiritualism and had become convinced that manipulation was the pathway to health. Billing himself throughout the 1880s as the "lightning bonesetter," Still traveled the disease circuit of Missouri in rumpled attire, setting hips and healing cripples in public squares to the amazement of gawking crowds.[53] In 1892, Still began teaching his system at the American School of Osteopathy in Kirksville, Missouri, three years before D.D. Palmer's first adjustment. Palmer was aware of Still's work and visited Kirksville on at least one occasion, though he claimed otherwise. Because Kirksville was only a day's journey for Palmer, it is unlikely that Palmer never traveled there. Further, Still's son Charles claimed that Palmer had stayed in his father's home, and several Missouri chiropractors reported seeing Palmer's name in Still's guestbook.[54]

The apparent similarity of technique between osteopathy and chiropractic left Palmer open to charges that his methods were simply a cheap imitation of Still's, a charge that Palmer continually denied, with considerable justification. Palmer's contention that he had never been in Kirksville probably arose from an intense desire to combat frequent charges from osteopaths that he had stolen chiropractic from Still. Although the spinal column was an area of special focus, Still held that disease resulted from an obstructed flow of bodily fluids, especially the blood. The obstruction was in turn caused by dislocated bones, particularly misalignments of vertebrae. While Palmer recognized "similar features" in the two methods, he insisted that chiropractic was unique because it was "founded upon the quality of nerve tissues and its [*sic*] ability to transmit functionating impulses," whereas osteopathy was founded upon the centrality of blood circulation. "Instead of nerves depending upon the arterial system for their quality of sensation, nutrition and motion, it is a fact, established by Chiropractic, that the arterial system depends upon the nervous system for the incentive stimulus which the latter possesses."[55] Palmer claimed too much—innovators are prone to exaggerations and to assertions of uniqueness and originality. But chiropractic was not simply osteopathy in new clothing. Palmer especially disliked Still's analogy of the body as a machine and the osteopath's acceptance of many allopathic notions. The basic difference in technique was that early osteopaths used different points of the body as fulcrums for bending and twisting, whereas chiropractors focused exclusively on the vertebrae, using the spinous and transverse processes as levers. There were important contrasts in theory and technique even though both originated from the same traditions.[56]

The bonesetting heritage, modernized by Still's osteopathy, aided the development of chiropractic by convincing Palmer of the value of drugless, "natural" techniques of manipulation. Palmer was sure that the bonesetters were on to something quite advanced and scientific, and the success of osteopaths boosted his confidence. In chiropractic, the soul cure of magnetic healing meshed with the hand cure of manipulation. Magnetic healing provided the vitalist, spiritualist path to chiropractic; the bonesetting tradition provided the practical, mechanical route. Palmer combined the two in developing his chiropractic system, a brash and cocksure synthesis that ensured that chiropractic would be ridiculed and shunned by the learned.

The "Science, Art and Philosophy" of Chiropractic

"What is life, disease, death and immortality?" posed D.D. Palmer. "These questions have been propounded by the savants of all ages and have remained unanswered until the advent of Chiropractic. This science and life are coexistent; it now answers the first three questions and in time will lift the veil which obstructs the view of the life beyond." In formulating his answers, Palmer began with the premise that an "All Wise" or "Universal Intelligence" ruled and permeated the universe, an intellect synonymous with "the Great Spirit, the Greek's Theos, the Christian's God, the Hebrew Helohim, the Mahometan's Allah, Hahneman's [sic] Vital Force, new thot's [thought's] Divine Spark, the Indian's Great Spirit, Hudson's Subconscious Mind, the Christian Scientist's All Goodness, the Allopath's Vis Medicatrix Naturae." Universal Intelligence finds personalized expression in being "metamerized," parceled into "metameres" required by each individual. This "Innate Intelligence," or simply *Innate* in Palmer's terminology, is a portion of the All Wise. Reminiscent of the Paracelsian Archeus, this "somatome" of the All is not subject to material laws, never sleeps, and is ever vigilant in caring for and directing bodily functions. Innate is "the conductor of life," which "superintends" the vital functions (innervation, circulation, transudation, respiration) and the vegetative functions (assimilation, growth, nutrition). Innate is the invincible master employing vital force and is not dependent upon the body that houses it, but becomes "associated with the physical" at baby's first breath. Innate is transmitted from the All Wise and not from the mother. In a metaphor later used by Palmer's son B.J., Universal Intelligence is the sun, Innate Intelligence the sunbeam.[57]

In addition to Innate, each individual possesses another intelligence that Palmer termed *Educated*. Unlike Innate, whose knowledge is eternal and not acquired, Educated is developed by the individual. Education and experience write upon the tabula rasa of Educated. Both Innate and Educated coexist in the same body, but Educated begins and ends with physical life. In contrast, Innate predates the body it inhabits and continues existence as an "individualized intelligence" beyond the life of the body, retaining for eternity information acquired by Educated. According to Palmer, Innate reasons by induction, from the particular to the general, while Educated proceeds by deduction, moving from general principles to a conclusion. Palmer never explained how an entity that begins as a blank slate could reason initially from general principles.

The power of Educated to garner experiential knowledge may be hindered by some defect of the bodily structure. A displacement of the osseous structure may press against a sensory nerve and distort the information that Educated receives and then transfers to Innate. The ability of Innate to pass to the life beyond full of useful experience depends upon the freedom of the "nerve channels of communication" to "convey the recognition of surrounding conditions and influences by which living forms are modified in their mental and physical growth."[58] The progression of life itself (spirit operating through matter) depends entirely upon the unobstructed communication of sensory impressions passing from the world to Educated to Innate through the nervous system.

Because the spine is the focal point of the nervous system, it stands as the crucial seat of this communications network. According to Palmer, ninety-five percent of all diseases are caused by displaced vertebrae, the rest by "luxations" of other joints. Displaced or "subluxated" vertebrae "impinge" on nerves, interfering with proper nerve transmission, creating a lack of ease, or "dis-ease." Nerve tension, "the condition of being tense, strained, stretched to stiffness, is the cause of all diseases; . . . normal tone is health." The specific disease depends upon which nerves are "too tense or too slack."[59]

But for Palmer, something much more is at stake than the physical well-being of the ailing individual—the march of Life is endangered when spinal subluxations go unadjusted. Innate, remarkable as it is in regulating body functions, providing healing power for broken bones, and channeling vital force, is incapable of adjusting displaced vertebrae. The chiropractor then intervenes to aid Innate. The chiropractor does not heal per se, but simply sets things aright so that proper bodily communication can resume. Akin to the alchemist, who believed that all metals would be gold but for the impurities of the earth, D.D. Palmer believed that all humans would be healthy but for the unnatural subluxations of the spine. Whereas the Philosopher's Stone of the alchemist was to turn a base metal into gold, transforming the imperfect to the most perfect of metals, the hands of the adept chiropractor would restore the imperfect, diseased body to its perfect and natural state of health. To Palmer, the chiropractor was much more than a mere body mechanic or back doctor. He was a philosophical scientist, a priest of Life, his healing hands the Philosopher's Stone.

In marrying magnetic healing to manipulation and emphasizing the centrality of nerve force[60] for the maintenance of health, Palmer believed that he had discovered not only the golden key to health, but also the pathway to life itself. D.D. Palmer's general vision was not the vision of a lone crank; that he considered his views to be scientific was not so unusual. His chiropractic philosophy was part of the harmonial tradition, a search for the Grand Principle of life which, unlike the mechanical approach that also sought monistic answers, expressed a need to integrate Spirit with Nature. Orthodox medicine had followed the dominant mechanical route, while the unorthodox approaches that developed in the eighteenth and nineteenth centuries frequently embraced the harmonial tradition. Until near the end of the nineteenth century all were searching for the Grand Principle, the orthodox (who often sought specific causes of disease as well) and the unorthodox alike. By the end of the century, however, the orthodox began discarding the pursuit of monisms that the unorthodox continued.[61] Palmer's panacea merely stood in a long line of monisms, as part of this elusive hunt for *the* cause of human ills. In its most reductionist form, the chiropractor simply located the subluxated vertebra that was impinging on a nerve and then adjusted it by hand. This emphasis on nerves as integral to physical life was nothing new. Scottish physician William Cullen (1712–90) had substituted the regulatory powers of the nervous system for the traditional humors in developing a general theory of health which held that debility was the product of a diminution of nervous energy and that spasm (the opposite of debility) came from an increase. Cullen's noted American student, Benjamin Rush, modified his mentor's theory by arguing that both a decrease *and* an increase in nervous energy resulted in debility. According to Rush this debility led to excitement, creating the opportunity for disease. Complaints of the patient were merely symptoms of a single disease, with different types of excitement acting upon a debility that already existed. Relieving the excitement through bloodletting and purging became the practical task of the physician.[62]

For Palmer, the practical task of the chiropractor became the adjustment of vertebrae to facilitate the flow of "nerve force." This prescription for health was an alluring, simple explanation. But such a simple answer to disease was anachronistic to medical men by the 1890s; for the learned, panaceas were passé.

For medical researchers, disease causation was now too complex to be reduced to a single, simplistic paradigm. *Legitimate complexity,* as medical sociologist Paul Starr termed it, was beginning to replace the popular notion engendered earlier in the century (especially by the Thomsonian movement) that causes and cures were simple matters within the grasp of Everyman. The growing authority of the medical profession was predicated largely upon public acceptance that health was a complex affair beyond the understanding of the layman and that it required the technical knowledge of a specialist who could demonstrate the material source of illness.[63] In contrast, D.D. Palmer offered his followers a scientific cosmology, an understanding of the world which tapped the optimistic, American version of the harmonial tradition, a view at odds with the notions of modern medical complexity. When science was shedding metaphysics at the end of the century and, in John Higham's phrasing, "the rational schemata . . . had become closed systems, imprisoning the human spirit," chiropractic became part of an impulse to reinvest science with spirit. According to Higham, the turn of the century brought a dynamic "reorientation of American culture," a spiritual reaction to the mechanization of life in numerous areas of popular culture. "To some of these areas," Higham argued, "historians have not yet paid enough attention to appreciate the extent and nature of the change that was occurring."[64]

One of these neglected fields which Higham himself failed to consider fully is a medical strain in the reorientation, especially the drugless therapy in popular medicine. Drugless therapy was a type of medical naturalism, the analogue of naturalist enthusiasm for vitality and the powers of nature apparent in such other areas of popular culture as sports and recreation, literature, and popular music. It is no mere coincidence that B.J. Palmer, son of D.D., became fast friends with Bernarr Macfadden, leading guru of the gospel of health and publisher of *Physical Culture,* a magazine that attracted a national audience. (Once, at a dinner B.J. attended in Macfadden's New York penthouse, Macfadden's three daughters danced artfully in the nude to no one's embarrassment, a tribute to naturalism and vital womanhood.)[65] With chiropractic, people conquer their illnesses by calling on Innate to overcome them, enlisting the powers of nature and healing without resorting to unnatural drugs. They return to the Source in order to heal.

Chiropractic prospered in large part because it joined the enthusiasm for nature's wonders and powers with a spiritual explanation of life and health. Chiropractic offered a middle way between the rationalism of the dominant science, which focused exclusively on Matter, and the drugless therapy of Christian Science, which focused entirely on Spirit. Chiropractic was a cosmology cast in the harmonial tradition, an integration of hand, heart, and mind. It was also a monistic answer that promised an escape from complexity and from specialization that constricted the spirit.

Unwittingly, however, chiropractic also benefited from the move toward medical specialization because it was easy to view chiropractors simply as back doctors, embued with special knowledge and techniques not available from orthodox physicians. Such a view frustrated Palmer, who saw himself as much more than a spine specialist with a limited range of usefulness. He believed that he had solved the mysteries of life and had developed a practical technique for alleviating the ills of humans. Yet, for back sufferers, the mysteries of life could often wait. Pain relief was the *critical* goal, and chiropractic offered relief from back ailments—administered by self-styled experts—that had eluded healers for generations. Chiropractic would gain adherents by easing back pain despite the protestations of D.D. Palmer that it involved much more. During the nineteenth century, neither self-help nor newer modes of treatment developed by physicians could conquer back ailments and attendant conditions. Such failure spelled opportunity for chiropractic.

Chapter Two

Of Doctor Books, Anodynes, and "Old Stubborn Pains in the Back" in Nineteenth-Century America

Every individual of the least penetration now claims the privilege of being his own physician:—it is not unfashionable to form a certain system concerning the state of our own health, and to consider it as the criterion, by which we may judge of ourselves and others, of patients, and their Physician.
James Parkinson, *The Town and Country Friend and Physician*

Study the nature of disease and how to remove it, and never trust your own life, nor that of a child, in the hands of what is called a family physician.
Samuel Thomson, *New Guide to Health or Botanic Family Physician*

Of the myriad pains that gnaw the human frame, none is more frustrating or debilitating than those related to the back and spine. In the nineteenth century, Americans battled lumbago and "the sciatica" (both considered to be specific forms of rheumatism) much as Americans wrestle with "slipped discs" and pinched nerves in the twentieth. Barring pain that results from violent injury, most back sufferers in both eras have probably attempted some sort of self-help before consulting a physician. "We frequently undertake the charge of prescribing medicines for ourselves," wrote Dr. James Parkinson in 1803, "and the natural consequence is, that we seldom are able to tell whether we are healthy or diseased; that we trust as much, if not more, to ourselves than to the Physician, who is only sent for occasionally." Malthus A. Ward, a frontier physician in western Pennsylvania and Indiana during the early nineteenth century, lamented that, even though influenza was prevalent, "the people believe it of no use to apply to a physician."[1] Such self-help in the twentieth century frequently begins with the aspirin bottle, but in the pre-aspirin age of the nineteenth it often began with the family "doctor book" or popular medical guide.

Doctor books have been perennial best sellers in America. The most popular in the eighteenth century was John Tennent's *Every Man his own Doctor: or, the Poor Planter's Physician*, first published in the second decade of the century and subsequently in numerous editions, the fourth in 1736 in Philadelphia, "re-printed and sold by B. Franklin, near the Market."[2] By the end of the 1700s, William Buchan's *Domestic Medicine; or the Family Physician*, published in Edinburgh in 1769 and continually printed in America until 1871, supplanted Tennent's work among the lay public.[3] During the last quarter of the nineteenth century, Ray Vaughn Pierce became the medical champion of the millions with *The People's Common Sense Medical Adviser in Plain English; or, Medicine Simplified*. First appearing in 1875, the *Adviser* apparently achieved the enviable combination of pertinent information and affordable price. The book sold over five million copies[4] and made Dr. Pierce (who also became a state senator of New York) a regional if not national celebrity. "Everyone who reads the newspapers," claimed the *New York Courier*, "has heard of Dr. R.V. Pierce, of Buffalo. . . . [His medical book] is of a size [over 900 pages] which generally sells for about $4.50 to $5.00, but the Doctor sells it for $1.50, and we do not know where a purchaser could expect to get so much really valuable information for so little money as in this hand-book."[5] Beginning "almost friendless, with no capital except his own manhood,"[6] Pierce's success enabled him to construct what he claimed was the largest sanitarium in the world, the Invalid's Hotel in Buffalo, which required a fifty dollar advance deposit as guarantee for "securing good apartments." Staffed by physicians and surgeons specializing in "chronic and lingering diseases," the sanitarium also offered free consultation by mail if the inquirers appended a list of acquaintances who were afflicted by chronic diseases. Pierce cautioned that, if the advisee sent a vial of urine for analysis, "a very small one will do, and all express charges on it must be prepaid."[7]

The doctor books written by Tennent, Buchan and Pierce were the most popular with the lay public, but dozens of others appeared during the course of the nineteenth century. Even before Pierce's *Adviser*, a good number of those who penned medical guides engaged in self-serving hucksterism, promoting themselves and their various medical wares with testimonials and recommendations while frequently insisting that their guides were being offered selflessly with considerable risk of censure by the medical profession for divulging the mysteries of the art. James Ewell, a distinguished southern physician who initiated vaccination in Savannah, wrote a popular guide used extensively in the South and West which went through ten editions in the early nineteenth century. Originally titled *The Planter's and Mariner's Medical Companion* (1807), it was dedicated to Thomas Jefferson, who had been an early classmate and companion of Ewell's father. Jefferson acknowledged the gift copy and dedication (reprinted in a preface along with dozens of other endorsements) by noting that the book "brings within a moderate compass whatever is useful, levels it to ordinary comprehension, and as a manual, will be a valuable possession to every family."[8] In an appendix complete with laudatory epistles from prominent medical and political friends, Ewell offered for public sale his carefully crafted and stocked "MEDICINE CHESTS," especially designed to accompany his guide. The chests contained scales and weights, mortar and pestle, spatula, lancets, syringes, injection pipes and bags, various plasters and ointments, and Epsom salts, as well as six rows of "handsomely labelled" bottles including opium, laudanum, ether, rheumatic tincture, "sirup" of squills, spirits of turpentine, solution of arsenic, oil of wormseed, "tooth-ach" drops, and elixir vitriol, among others. "Thus making an assortment of Medicines," asserted Ewell, "sufficiently complete as to furnish an appropriate remedy for every disease. The author also warrants them to be genuine, and it will be found that his price is below the retail prices in any city of the United States." His price for such peace of mind was "a moderate" fifty dollars if the customer was willing to settle for a chest made of "mock mahogany." For chests made of cherry wood "with double flint glass and ground stopper bottles," the price grew to seventy-five dollars and, for "elegant mahogany cases, with glass stopper bottles of much larger size," the cost was one hundred dollars, double that of the basic model. Apparently sales were brisk. Ewell felt compelled to warn potential purchasers that, because the reputation of his chests had "aroused the spirit of imposters, Dr. E. feels it his duty to inform the Public, that in future his agents will carry certificates with the seal of Washington annexed."[9]

This same combination of duty-bound selflessness and self-promotion was evident in the 1837 offering of J.A. Brown entitled *The Family Guide to Health*. In his concluding remarks, Brown suggested that "it may be incumbent on the author to offer his readers something in the form of an apology. The undertaking was not induced, either by love of notoriety, or of book-making, or the hope of gain." In the next few pages, however, Brown was ready to present his services to the reader by offering a stock of family medicine since "there are but few who have either the opportunity or inclination to search the fields and forests for these productions." The medicines could be purchased individually, but those who bought all at the same time (for five dollars) would receive a copy of his book, gratis, "and to those who may not wish for the book, a proportionate discount will be made, provided they shall have previously obtained one." Brown also proposed "an enlarged and improved form" of the *Guide* for a price of five dollars "to be put to press as soon as one hundred responsible subscribers shall have been obtained."[10]

Some authors of doctor books were much less circumspect about expressing a desire for profit and made little pretense of altruism. William Daily of Louisville, Kentucky, in *The Indian Doctor's Practice of Medicine. Daily's Family Physician* (1848), purposely withheld inclusion of the ingredients of two compounds, one for dysentery and the other his patented "Pain Extractor." The price of the book was too low, according to Daily, "to have so great a discovery revealed—a discovery that has cost me seven years labor and research." He was quite willing, however, to part with a bottle for one dollar, complete with a promise that a single tablespoonful would effect a cure. For his patented revelation, Daily concocted a type of franchise scheme. "I will sell the exclusive right to make and vend my *Magic Drops* or *Pain Extractor* for States, Counties, Cities, or Parishes, for a reasonable compensation," he offered, "to be regulated according to location, population, etc. Those within the limits of my practice need not apply." Inquiries for particulars would be answered if postage was paid. "Now is the time to make a fortune," Daily proclaimed, concluding with the afterthought, "and to save thousands from an early grave."[11]

Perhaps the strangest doctor book of the midnineteenth century combined white magic with Christian mysticism. Compiled by John George Hohman and titled *The Long Lost Friend or Faithful & Christian Instructions Containing Wondrous and Well-Tried Arts & Remedies, for Man as Well as Animals* (1850), it suggested remedies for everything from "Hysterics, (or Mother-Fits)" to consumption to rheumatism. In addition, Hohman offered advice for making hens lay eggs, causing thieves to stand still, preventing witches from bewitching cattle, making wands to search for iron or water, and winning every game of cards, and he even included "effective benedictions" for use against worms and other assorted enemies and pests. In detailing his reasons for publishing the book, Hohman was self-congratulatory and stated baldly his financial motives.

> And I therefore ask thee again, oh friend, male or female, is it not to my everlasting praise, that I have had such books printed? Do I not deserve the rewards of God for it? Where else is the physician that could cure these diseases? Besides that, I am a poor man, in needy circumstances, and it is a help to me if I can make a little money with the sale of my books.[12]

Most people who consulted a doctor book, however, were probably little interested in the motives of the author. Only those who competed directly for the medical attentions of the public seem to have raised an outcry against the guides. "As was expected, frightful symptoms of discomfiture appeared among all the *penny-wise* venders and dispensers of drugs," explained William M. Hand in a preface to the second edition (1820) of *The House Surgeon and Physician,* "which reminds one of the shrieking and scampering of the witches, when an honest guest said grace at their table."[13] Orthodox members of the medical profession also raised opposition to the guides as well as the nostrum vendors condemned by Hand. The *New York Medical Repository,* in reviewing James Ewell's *Medical Companion,* clarified the protest of medical men.

> Manuals of health, or popular publications on medicine, have become so frequent as to have excited the censure of some grave and oracular members of the profession. They consider their publishing brethren as unnecessarily divulging the arcana of the art, as deprecating its credit and estimation, and as teaching the common mass of readers to know as much as themselves. This communicative disposition they conceive to be carried to a very faulty extreme. For when the secrets of the healing faculty are promulgated by its members, with such consummate knowledge and success, what is left from distinguishing the regularly initiated from those who are without the pale? The propagation of the Esculapian mysteries is viewed to be faulty on another account; in as much as in diminishing the importance, it lessens the profits of the practisers, and thus, for the gratification and emolument of one telltale author, the whole fraternity is disparaged.[14]

The medical laity who thumbed the doctor books for help were probably as little interested in the internecine struggles of the medical fraternity as they were in the author's pecuniary motives. Most were willing to grant the writers a moderate profit as long as the remedies found within the books relieved them of pain. How did the authors address the ubiquitous backache that undoubtedly sent many to the guides? What types of anodynes (pain relievers) and treatments did the writers prescribe for back pain before the age of aspirin, acetaminophen, and ibuprofen?[15]

Pain in the back is mentioned as one of the "signs discovering the Assault" of smallpox in the earliest medical document printed in America. *A Brief Rule to guide the Common-People of New-England how to order themselves and theirs in the Small Pocks, or Measels* by the Reverend Thomas Thacher was issued as a broadside dated "21. 11. 1677/8" (January 21, 1677/78) and was aimed at the lay public.[16] Thacher was, of course, much more concerned with eradicating the pustules and fevers associated with the pox than with attendant conditions such as back pain. This document does suggest, however, an awareness that back pain could result from a host of problems not principally related to the back.

The first domestic medical book published in America was also by a minister-physician, the famous John Wesley. His *Primitive Physick: or, an Easy and Natural Method of Curing Most Diseases* was a "classic do-it-yourself medical book" published in thirty-two English and seven American editions between 1747 and 1829.[17] It was reprinted more frequently than any of Wesley's religious offerings and probably reached a wider reading public.[18] *Primitive Physick* was compiled in a style reminiscent of scripture. The various ailments corresponded to numbered chapter divisions, and alternative methods of treating each problem corresponded to verses (but were numbered consecutively throughout the book). Often domestic medical authors included back problems as a particular form of rheumatism or under an entry labeled sciatica. Wesley included separate prescriptions for each of these problems, and those who searched the various guides for back relief certainly considered using possibilities listed under all three as well as concoctions recommended as general anodynes. Wesley's ailment number 147, "An old Stubborn Pain in the Back," was treated by steeping "root of Water-Fern in Water, till the Water becomes thick and clammy. Then rub the Parts therewith Morning and Evening."[19] Entry 164, "The Rheumatism," suggested numerous alternatives:

536 Use the *Cold Bath*, with Rubbing and Sweating:
537 Or, rub in warm *Treacle* [molasses], and apply to the Part a brown Paper smeared therewith: Change it twelve Hours:
538 Or, drink very largely of warm Water in Bed:
539 Or, *Tar-water* Morning and Evening:
540 Or, steep six or seven Cloves of *Garlick* in half a Pint of white Wine. Drink it lying down. It sweats and frequently cures at once:
541 Or, mix flour of *Brimstone* with *Honey*, equal Quantyties. Take three Tea-spoonfuls at Night, two in the Morning; and one afterwards Morning and Evening, till cured. This succeeds oftener than any Remedy I have found:
542 Or, take Morning and Evening as much *Lignum Guaiacum* powder'd, as lies on a Shilling:
543 Or, as much *Flour of Sulphur*, washing it down with a Decoction of *Lignum Guaiacum:*
544 Or, live on *new Milk Whey* and *white Bread* for fourteen Days. This has cured in a desparate Case.[20]

"The Sciatica," defined by Wesley as "a violent Pain in the Hip, chiefly in the Joint of the Thigh Bone," was complaint number 174. He suggested a purging quickly after an attack, cold bathing and sweating used with the "Flesh Brush" twice a day, drinking half a pint of cold water in the morning and at four in the afternoon, daily for four to five days, applying "bruised" ranunculus (buttercup) leaves and the "pounded roots" of burdock and elicompane, administering a poultice of boiled nettles fomented with liquor, drinking a "decoction" of boiled calamint and also applying it externally as a poultice, and dipping flannels in stale lye boiled with salt, applying them "as hot as you can bear, for an hour."[21]

Unlike many of the authors who first published in the nineteenth century, Wesley was wary of strong drugs and excessive bloodletting for pain relief, aversions that undoubtedly contributed to the popularity of his manual.[22] "It is because they are not safe, but extremely dangerous, that I have omitted (together with Antimony) the four *Herculian* Medicines, Opium, the [Peruvian] Bark, Steel, and the various Preparations of Quick-silver," Wesley explained. "Herculian indeed! Far too strong for common Men to grapple with. How many fatal Effects have these produced, even in the Hands of no ordinary Physicians?"[23]

John Tennent (*Every Man His Own Doctor*) echoed Wesley's sentiments but made it clear that reticence in recommending strong drugs was unusual.

> It may seem strange, that, among the Remedies I have prescrib'd, no mention is made of *Mercury, Opium,* or the *Peruvian Bark,* which have almost obtain'd the Reputation of *Specificks.* I acknowledge the powerful Effects of these Medicines; but am perswaded, they ought to be administered with the greatest Skill, and Discernment. And, as I write chiefly for the Service of the Poor who are wholly left to judge for themselves, I was fearful of putting such dangerous Weapons into their Hands.[24]

By the nineteenth century the doctor books were much less guarded about strong drugs and cautioned against excessive usage rather than advocating abstention. Two popular, contradictory beliefs regarding the efficacy of drugs underscored the deficiency of theoretical understanding. Some believed that drugs cured through nonspecific physiological properties as cathartics or emetics, while others held that a particular drug was specific to a particular disease.[25] Regardless of viewpoint, opium was becoming the drug of choice for general pain relief.[26] John C. Gunn in *Gunn's Domestic Medicine* (first published in 1807) touted the poppy extract as "the monarch of medicinal powers, the soothing angel of moral and physical pain." Unlike wine or spirits, which "unsettle and cloud the judgment," opium

> produces a just equipose between our intellectual strength and sensibilities; arouses all our dormant faculties; and disposes them to harmonious and pleasurable activity; and with regard to the temper, moral energies, and physical sensations in general, opium produces that sort of simple and vital animation, that cordial warmth of feeling and sensibility which we would almost suppose to have accompanied man in his primeval and unfallen state.

After such a breathless commendation, Gunn's insistence that opium be used only for its medicinal qualities "as intended by the Great Father of the universe" and not as a stimulant or luxury rang hollow. Gunn even lamented the fact that Americans were spending huge annual sums for opium which served only to enrich foreigners. He suggested that southern and western states had the proper climate and soil to allow cultivation of quantities sufficient for the needs of all Americans and gave explicit and detailed directions on planting and cultivating techniques.[27]

Those who consulted such doctor books would likely employ opium in its various forms (as laudanum, paregoric, and morphine or in mixtures such as Bateman's elixir,[28] Godfrey's cordial, and Dover's powder) for back pain. According to Gunn, opium was combined more frequently "with more medicines for the cure of diseases than any other drug known to or used by medical men. In every patent medicine sold in the shops, especially for the relief of pain in diseases, opium forms the principal portion."[29] By the nineteenth century opium was prescribed freely for pain relief by orthodox medical advisors as long as moderate doses were administered.[30] Unorthodox medical sects such as the Thomsonians, however, balked at administering such "poisons as medicine" and gained a large following by offering nontoxic botanic remedies. Likewise the homeopaths, led by German physician Samuel Hahnemann, reacted by prescribing infinitesimal doses based on the principle of *similai similibus curantur* (let likes be cured by likes)—that illness could be cured by substances that produced the same symptoms in a healthy person manifested by those who were sick.[31]

In addition to embracing strong drugs more easily than did their eighteenth-century predecessors, early nineteenth-century domestic medical writers also much more readily endorsed bloodletting and its corollary techniques of cupping and leeching. Bloodletting as a universal remedy for disease was championed principally by Dr. Benjamin Rush. After some success in treating yellow fever patients by bloodletting during the epidemic of 1793, Rush concluded that all fevers and, by extension, all diseases resulted from excessive tension in the blood vessels. This sole cause of disease had a sole remedy—relieve the pressure. The lancet would let blood, while mighty emetics and cathartics such as calomel (mercurous chloride) would purge the stomach and bowels.[32]

Undergirding these "heroic" practices lay a set of deeply held assumptions common to both practitioners and laymen; these assumptions provided a rational framework with a pedigree dating from classical antiquity. In the early nineteenth century, the notion that the body was a living system in constant and dynamic interaction with its environment was the prevailing metaphor that explained the body's general state of health and disease. Acting in concert, heredity and environment determined physical well-being at any given time. Environmental circumstances such as climate, style of work, and the intake of air, food, and water were in continual flux and forced the body into perpetual adjustments, always in a position of becoming and therefore always in peril.

In addition, common wisdom linked every part of the body intimately to every other. For example, an upset stomach could easily create mental confusion; conversely, a troubled mind could convulse the stomach. Similarly, systemic ailments could cause or be caused by local sores—all bodily features, whether local or systemic, were interconnected. The body was a system of inflow and outflow, and health resulted from a proper balance of the two. Customary admonitions on proper diet, evacuation, and perspiration were rooted in this understanding. Equilibrium meant health; disequilibrium meant illness. The physician sought to "regulate the secretions" (extracting blood or inducing urination, for example) and thereby aid the body in regaining its normal balance.[33]

Alexander Thomson (no relation to Samuel or to the Thomsonian movement) in *The Family Physician* (1802), following Rush's lead and steeped in these commonplace medical assumptions, prescribed bleeding for "all topical inflammations of internal parts" and for "local fixed pain," which would include back pain.[34] Such an operation, Thomson assured, could be performed easily by those "without professional education . . . where the assistance of a surgeon cannot readily be obtained."[35] Bleeding should be performed with a lancet as near as possible to the affected part; if a vein was unavailable, however, leeching or cupping would be necessary.

Thomson gave explicit instructions to the home novice on the proper application of leeches. Before attaching them,

> the skin should be carefully cleaned from any foulness, and moistened with a little milk, by which means they fasten more readily, and this farther promoted by allowing them to creep upon a dry cloth, or a dry board, for a few minutes before application. The most effectual method to make them fix upon a particular spot, is to confine them to the part by means of a small wine glass. As soon as the leeches have separated, the useful method of promoting the discharge of blood is, to cover the parts with fine linen cloths wet in warm water. But if the blood should continue to flow from the orifice made by a leech, longer than is desired, as has happened in some instances, to children, who have been nearly lost by the inability of the attendants to stop the discharge; after carefully washing off the blood, the point of the finger should be pressed moderately upon the orifice, and afterwards a compress should be kept upon it for a little time.

In addition to leeches, Thomson also explained that scarification and cupping could be used when it was deemed necessary to "evacuate blood" directly from the vessels of the affected part. "Slight scarifications" could be made by using the edge or shoulder of a lancet or by a specially constructed instrument dubbed a "scarificator; in which fifteen or twenty lancets are commonly placed, in such a manner that when the instruments is [*sic*] applied to the part affected, the whole number of lancets contained in it are, by means of a strong spring, pushed suddenly into it, to the depth at which the instrument has been previously regulated." Such a process did not promote the free discharge of blood since only the small vessels were cut. Specially constructed cupping glasses, designed with a small hole in the bottom, were often fitted over the scarified part. The attendant would enhance blood flow by placing his mouth over the cup and creating suction or by an improvement called an "exhausting syringe" which facilitated extraction of air from the cups. The application of heat to the cupping glasses (to "rarefy the air" for producing sufficient suction) was Thomson's technique of choice, since it was difficult to maintain air-tight suction with the syringe. If the discharge of blood still proved insufficient, the scarificator and cupping glasses would need to be reapplied as close to the former site as possible. An alternate procedure dubbed *dry cupping*, the application of the cupping glasses without the scarificator, produced a tumor over the affected part and was advised "where any advantage is to be expected from a determination of blood to a particular part."[36]

Bleeding was a necessary treatment, according to Thomson, for both acute and chronic rheumatism, the former distinguished by an accompanying fever. After bleeding from a vein, six or eight leeches could be attached to the "tumefied parts" on two successive days to "great advantage." Gentle purgatives and sudorifics (medicines that promote perspiration) were judged second only to bloodletting in effectiveness. Strong drugs such as Dover's powder, nitre "joined with" antimony, the Peruvian bark, and calomel combined with opium were suggested as efficacious remedies, as were both cold bathing (particularly in salt water) and warm bathing.

Specifically for lumbago (pain in the lower or lumbar region of the spine), Thomson offered two quite different possibilities. The first was the use of "issues." These were artificially induced ulcers, purposely formed to procure "a discharge of purulent matter" and considered to be therapeutic for a variety of disorders by draining "noxious humours" from the blood. By the early 1800s, the quantity of purulent matter induced was held to be the most important curative factor and supplanted the former notion that placement of the issues close to the affected part was the primary concern. Because pus over placement had become the medical watchword, issues were installed where they were least inconvenient to the afflicted. They could be located "wherever there is a sufficiency of cellular substance for the protection of the parts beneath." Spots that met these qualifications, according to Thomson, were "the nape of the neck; the middle, outer, and fore part of the shoulder; the hollow above the inner side of the knee; or either side of the backbone; or between two of the ribs." For lumbago, he specifically recommended the leg or thigh, whereas the arm was the proper place if the upper parts were affected.

The issues in common usage were the blister issue, the pea issue, and the seton or cord issue. In the first type, heat or caustics applied to the chosen spot created a blister. The blister was removed, and pus was kept flowing by daily dressing with an ointment of cantharides (dried and powdered Spanish flies), which acted as a skin irritant. Discharge could be regulated by the application of a milder irritant or by using the cantharides less frequently.

A pea issue was formed by thrusting one or more peas (kidney beans, gentian root, or orange peas were possible substitutes) into an incision made by a lancet or an opening caused by a caustic substance. The peas chafed the wound and created the necessary secretion.

The seton or cord issue (cord to be composed of cotton or silk threads) was used when large quantities were desired, "especially from deep-seated parts." When the cord was introduced into the body, Thomson directed that "the parts at which it is to enter and pass out should be previously marked with ink; and a small part of the cord being besmeared with some mild ointment, and passed through the eye of the seton-needle, the part is to be supported by an assistant, and the needle passed fairly through, leaving a few inches of the cord hanging out." The degree of irritation was regulated by the type of ointment applied to the cord, to be repeated daily until sufficient quantity was produced.

Thomson's other remedy for lumbago was much more likely to please a back sufferer than the use of issues. To two drams of camphor dissolved in two drams of oil of turpentine, the afflicted should add an ounce of basilicon, a half-ounce of common black soap, and half a dram of volatile sal ammoniac. The mixture was to be spread on leather and applied to the lower back.

Thomson's concoction, however, was only one entry in a parade of curatives. Poultices, cataplasms, and plasters were commonly prescribed for back pain in the doctor books of the nineteenth century and often echoed prescriptions given in the eighteenth. James Ewell in his *Medical Companion* (1807) gave the recipe for a multipurpose mixture that had gained some reputation as a specific for back pain. It is based on what is probably the same plant described much earlier by Wesley as the Water-fern and touted as a treatment for an "old stubborn pain in the back." Labeled by Ewell as "Fern Female or Backach Brake," it

> grows near ponds, and in moist pastures, about twelve inches high. The leaves are single, winged, and about a hand's length; the root is about the size of a goose quill, of a brown colour, very sweet, and of a mucilaginous taste.
>
> A quart of a strong decoction of the roots, and a pint of honey, formed into a sirup, by gentle simmering and given in doses of a table-spoonful every hour or two, is esteemed highly beneficial in all violent coughs. It is said that three parts of the roots of this plant, and one part of sumach root, boiled slowly in any kind of spirits, until it becomes slimy, and then applied warm to the spine, has frequently relieved the backach; hence the vulgar name, backach brake. It has also been employed as a remedy for the rickets in children.[37]

J.A. Brown in *The Family Guide to Health* (1837) divulged ingredients for a "strengthing plaster" that included components suggested by previous writers. The plaster was "a very good preparation to apply to the back, or other parts of the body, affected with weakness" and consisted of burdock and mullen leaves combined with enough turpentine and rosin to give it the proper consistency to spread on leather. Brown also recommended the cold application of a cure-all poultice of powdered crackers, ginger, and slippery elm bark moistened with coffee.[38]

In addition to the numerous preparations described in doctor books intermittently throughout the 1800s,[39] by midcentury health watchers touted the curative powers of water for back ailments and associated pains. The "water cure," the internal and external application of "pure water," was an ancient method revived in the United States by the eighteenth century and elevated to scientific status by the midnineteenth. It represented a therapeutically conservative movement away from harsh bleedings and purgings. Hydropathic institutes dotting the countryside offered drugless water therapy combined with a temperate diet and moderate exercise. These establishments held a special appeal for women by allowing them a legitimate escape from the isolated sick rooms of home to the comradery of a largely female-oriented environment where attention to exercise, message, and bathing offered sensual experiences not often available to the respectable middle-class woman.[40] American women apparently needed such retreats from both physical and psychological standpoints. Catharine Beecher, sister of Harriet Beecher Stowe and Henry Ward Beecher and stalwart advocate of domesticity for women, sampled the state of female health in seventy-nine communities in the mid-nineteenth century and reported, in *Letters to the People on Health and Happiness* (1855), a three-to-one ratio of sick to healthy.[41]

One of the numerous and nagging female debilitations was back pain. The strain of childbearing translated into chronic backache and represented a perennial problem for women. Demands of culture and sophistication also contributed considerably to the ailment. The fashionable urban woman cut a wasp-waisted figure, gathering in the excess by tight-lacing herself in a whalebone corset. During winter months, her street garb averaged thirty-seven pounds, nineteen of which cascaded from the waist. This load, in combination with the corseting (which put extraordinary pressures on the spinal column, displaced internal organs, collapsed lungs, and caused "chicken-breasts"—an overlapping of the ribs that created labored breathing and injured the sternum and clavicle), guaranteed unremitting back troubles.[42] Even a self-assured sadist would be hard pressed to devise a more ingenious method of inducing lumbar pain in the stylish woman.

The water cure, taken at a hydropathic institute, promised relief and freed women temporarily from the strictures of tight-lacing. Catherine

Beecher's quest for personal health led her to temporary residence at thirteen different water-cure spas. In the waning days of her life, she went to live in Elmira, New York, to be close to its hydropathic establishment. Water, according to Beecher, could work wonders on the back. In an appendix to her *Letters*, she endorsed a communication written by "Mrs. Dr." R.B. Gleason of the Elmira Water Cure.

It is probable that thousands of women who are suffering from pain in the back and pelvic evils, and who either soon will be invalids or imagine themselves so, could be relieved entirely by obeying these directions:

1. Wash the whole person on rising in cool water. Dress loosely, and let *all* the weight of clothing rest on the shoulders.
2. Sleep in a well-ventilated room; exercise the muscles a great deal, especially those of the arms and trunk, taking care to lie down and rest as soon as fatigue is felt.
3. Take a sitting-bath ten minutes at a time, in the middle of the forenoon and afternoon with water at 85, reducing it gradually each day till at 60. Let the water reach above the hip, and while bathing rub and press the abdomen *upward*.

Wear a double girdle by night around the lower part of the body. Make it one-third of a yard wide; wring it well, and when on, cover it with double cotton flannel. If pain and weakness are felt, wear it by day also, adding clothing enough to prevent chilliness.[43]

J. Cam Massie also lauded the curative powers of water in his 1854 offering titled *Treatise on the Eclectic Southern Practice of Medicine*. He recommended the application of the "wet sheet" dipped in weak lye as an "indispensable remedy" for "the treatment of most of our diseases." The reader could interpret the sheet as providing relief from backache, since Massie claimed it "to be the most soothing application that can be administered to the external sentient surface. It may in effect be compared to a soothing poultice placed over some portion of the body." For treating rheumatic problems, Massie suggested a variation called the "alcoholic vapor bath" as being especially successful. The patient was wrapped in a blanket and placed in a "solid bottomed chair" with feet immersed in warm water. The patient sipped "freely of some diaphoretic tea" while alcohol was heated in an open saucer under the chair. When fatigued the patient was to be wrapped tightly in the blanket, placed in bed and allowed to perspire "for some length of time." The attendant then rubbed the patient with lye and dried him to the pink of health with a coarse towel.[44]

Beecher, Massie, and others who embraced the tenets of hydropathy offered the various modes of the water cure as a specific alternative to the lancet, an alternative that avoided the loss of strength and general debility occasioned by the heroic measures. Another feature of this growing medical conservatism adopted by many water advocates was the medical use of electricity.[45] After midcentury, evolving theories on the nature of the nervous system suggested a therapeutic use for electricity. In 1869, physician George M. Beard coined the term *neurasthenia* to explain the nervous exhaustion or "nervelessness" he believed endemic in the middle classes of urban America, caused by the increased use of "brain force" which marked the evolutionary price paid by an advancing civilization. Symptoms were vague and protean, running the gamut from spinal irritation to "flying neuralgias" to "fidgetiness" to ticklishness. Explanations of the mental and physical breakdown neurasthenia wrought tended to be metaphorical—a small furnace with little fuel that fired too quickly, an overdrawn bank account, a spent battery, an overloaded electrical circuit. Physicians commonly believed that each individual held a fixed quantity of nerve force or energy, dictated mainly by heredity, which animated the various parts of the body. When demand outstripped supply, nervous exhaustion resulted. For example, overwork, excessive worry, or inadequate food or rest could trigger an acute attack or create chronic exhaustion. In an updated version of common wisdom from earlier in the century, stress on one system, such as overworking the brain, could cause the digestive or reproductive system harm through the principle of reflex irritation and could initiate a total bodily breakdown.[46]

The intemperate expenditure of energy by the nervous system was attributed to a defect in the molecular makeup of the protoplasm of gray "neurine" cells; this defect caused the protoplasm to disintegrate faster than the body could repair it. *Neurenergen,* as coined by Sanger Brown of Chicago, described the form of nervous energy that organic matter took as it converted itself for bodily use. Health meant a continual flow of neurenergen current into the neurons, ready for use as needed. The neurons of the neurasthenic, however, malfunctioned and were unable to maintain a proper quantity of neurenergen. Given this understanding, physicians logically discussed nervous activity in electrical terms and often compared the brain and nervous system to a galvanic battery whose duty was to deliver a steady, dependable flow of current or "special fluid" for consumption. Application of electricity to the body became an attempt to restore "conductibility" to the neuron, inducing proper transmission of nerve impulses.[47]

Emerging views on the application of electricity affected how the layman was counseled to deal with back and spinal problems. Dr. Frederick Hollick, in his immodestly titled *The Family Physician; or, the True Art of Healing the Sick in All Diseases Whatever* (1851), insisted that old methods of treating spinal malfunctions were not only outmoded but actually harmful to the patient. As one example he cited the case of a seventeen-year-old woman whose spine had only a slight curve from the perpendicular but nonetheless she "had suffered some pretty strong treatment by cups and tartar emetic ointment, till her back was one mass of scars, but still was no stronger, which, indeed was hardly to be wondered at, for such treatment is more likely to *cause* weakness than to *remove* it." Instead, he had administered galvanic treatments designed to stimulate muscle activity, typically accomplished by passing electric current through the body with two conductors (often covered with wet linen) attached to a battery. Hollick claimed a successful and enduring cure. "In a short time after applying the battery," Hollick reported the patient standing with posture erect and no further complaints of pain or weakness. The old methods of blistering, cupping, leeching, and covering the back with issues should be abandoned, Hollick reasoned, since "it is more than probable that when a recovery takes place under such treatment, it is rather in spite of it than by its means." He also held that the galvanic battery could successfully treat a host of problems, including dyspepsia, constipation, consumption, asthma, neuralgia, paralysis, tumors, female diseases, and sterility.[48]

Along with the growing avoidance of the old heroic measures, doctor books continued to recommend homespun remedies reminiscent of concoctions promoted earlier in the century. Isaac Shinn in *The Ready Advisor and Family Guide* (1866) suggested that those affected with the various forms of rheumatism should try, among other things, bathing the affected part in water in which potatoes had been boiled, drinking poke berries in brandy every day for three weeks, eating asparagus and Jerusalem artichokes, and imbibing a mixture of pipsissewa (wintergreen) and pure rye whiskey.[49] George Beard (*Our Home Physician,* 1869), reflecting the developing theories on nerve force, exhibited a more sophisticated understanding of back ailments by recognizing backache as "a *symptom* of numberless diseases" and by understanding the role of nerves issuing from the spine as central to much back pain, creating what he called "headache in the back." Beard believed that the majority of backaches could be attributed to "nervous exhaustion" (what he would later dub neurasthenia) and that pain in the "small of the back" was frequently caused by dyspepsia or "derangement of the digestive organs." Less frequently, according to Beard, diseases of the genital organs, spine and spinal cord, and kidneys caused back pain, whereas the principal fevers of the era—smallpox and remittent, intermittent, and yellow fever—were "ushered in by pain in the back."[50]

Despite this greater theoretical understanding and his insistence that the *cause* must be treated, Beard had nothing really new to offer the sufferer in this particular book. For general backache he recommended the decades-old "anodyne plasters" and various liniments and for lumbago the antiquated method of dry cupping and the use of "spongio-piline," an "extemporaneous poultice" made of rubber and lined with a quarter-inch of sponge and wool that was little more than an updated version of the midcentury wet sheet.[51]

Soon, however, Beard was touting the curative powers of electricity in *A Practical Treatise on the Medical and Surgical Uses of Electricity* (1881), which gave explicit instructions to practitioners on the application of electrical power for ailments of all varieties. But such treatment required visiting a physician. For those who desired electrical self-help, "Dr. Scott's Electric FLESH Brush," as advertised in *Harper's Weekly* in October 1881, was "WARRANTED TO CURE . . . rheumatism and Diseases of the Blood, Nervous Complaints, Neuralgia, Toothache, Malarial, Lameness, Palpitation, Paralysis, and ALL pains caused by Impaired circulation" and promised promptly to alleviate indigestion, liver and kidney troubles, and those " 'Back Aches' peculiar to Ladies," while imparting "wonderful vigor to the whole body." This three dollar marvel ("Not a Wire Brush but Pure Bristles") used a new, ebony-like material for its back which produced a "permanent Electro Magnetic Current" and could always be tested for potency by a silver compass that accompanied each brush. The brush worked, according to the advertisement, "because it quickens the circulation, opens the pores, and enables the system to throw off those impurities which cause disease." Daily use would impart "New Energy and New Life" as well as "A Beautiful Clear Skin" by acting instantly upon the blood, nerves, and tissues. A motto carved on the back assured the user that "The Germ of all Life is Electricity."[52]

By the end of the century, Dr. R.V. Pierce of Buffalo, New York, was offering something novel, without electricity, for the chronic back sufferer; this new device echoed the American fascination with mechanical gadgets. In a section labeled "Mechanical Aids in the Cure of Chronic Diseases" in *The People's Common Sense Medical Adviser,* Pierce described the operation of "The Manipulator," which he used at his Invalids' Hotel. The device consisted of several wheels of varying sizes which could transmit motion vertically, horizontally, and diagonally with suitable attachments. The Manipulator transformed "mechanical into vital energy, thereby restoring strength to the feeble and helpless." It was used to rub the back, arms and legs, chest, and abdomen and to oscillate the arms and legs. The action of the Manipulator resembled that of the "living operator" but was much more efficient, according to Pierce, because it was "impossible for the unaided hand to impart the degree of rapidity necessary to secure the effects easily obtained by the machine."[53] Efficiency, increasingly the watchword for America's emerging industrial economy, was also being touted as a key for curing America's sick. Perhaps it took such vigorous stimulation to make a physical impression on Americans increasingly oriented to a fast-paced industrial workplace. Walter Rauschenbusch, noted liberal minister and reformer, commented that "the long hours and the high speed and pressure of industry use up the vitality of all except the most capable. An exhausted body craves rest, change, and stimulus, but it responds only to strong and coarse stimulation."[54] Yet people respond positively to the human touch when seeking relief from pain.[55] Both in industry and on the farm, work was increasingly mechanized; Americans would be likely to react against being treated by a machine when seeking relief from ailments such as back pain, which traditionally had been cared for by more personal methods. A conservative curative approach offering demonstrable pain relief which could combine the human touch with "strong and coarse stimulation" would probably be able to carve out a considerable niche for itself in the healing community.

The opportunity for an alternative mode was also enhanced by the fact that no definitive treatment for back problems emerged during the century. The doctor books of the nineteenth century proffered such an array of advice for back ailments that the average reader was likely to be more confused than helped. "It is notorious," wrote Dr. Frederick Hollick, "that medical treatment scarcely ever does so [arrest spinal deformity], and hardly any two practitioners advise the same course with it." Dr. John King in *The American Family Physician; or, Domestic Guide to Health* (1892) confessed that, although spinal problems were very common, "the treatment generally pursued for spinal disease is not attended with any great amount of success, for the very reason that it is debilitating in its character, as every one knows who has witnessed its treatment by emetics, cathartics, blisters, etc."[56] Even the novel and usually more conservative treatments (such as hydropathy and galvanism) had failed to alleviate the pain of the multitude of back sufferers.[57] Dr. R.V. Pierce noted the obstinancy of acute rheumatism, which often "resists for many days the best treatment yet known to the medical profession." Pierce also expressed his exasperation at attempting to instruct the layman in the treatment of chronic rheumatism. "I frankly acknowledge my inability to so instruct the non-professional reader as to enable him to detect the various systemic faults common to this ever-varying disease, and adjust remedies to them, so as to make the treatment uniformly successful." If self-treatment was unsuccessful, Pierce advised the reader to consult the expert physician.[58]

By the end of the century the failure of self-help for back ailments was evident. The newer modes of treatment (such as the galvanic battery and the mechanical manipulator) could not be easily self-administered; the sufferer had to depend on the skill of a self-styled expert for relief. The populace wanted conservative therapy, but those offered to date had failed to provide sufficient relief for the plague of back pain in its various forms. There was, then, both a failure of self-help and a failure of professional help regarding back pain and related spinal problems. The "expert" was being lauded in most fields, but the emerging medical experts could do little for the back sufferer—the promise of pain relief was largely a chimera. For thousands, the reality of excruciating back pain continued to surpass the promises of relief. Those with old stubborn pains in the back were ready for conservative yet active treatment that retained the human touch.

Chiropractors themselves stood ready to fill this physical need. In ministering to this need, however, it was quite possible to ignore the spiritual component of D.D. Palmer's system and embrace only the theory of disease or the techniques of adjustment. Palmer offered an answer to life, but his integration of Spirit and Nature could easily be stripped of Spirit and suffer few practical consequences. Disagreements over what constituted true chiropractic widened the schisms that would wrack the chiropractic world.

Chapter Three

The Chiropractic Kaleidoscope

A company of porcupines crowded themselves very close together one cold winter's day so as to profit by one another's warmth and so save themselves from being frozen to death. But soon they felt one another's quills, which induced them to separate again. And now, when the need for warmth brought them nearer together again, the evil arose once more. So that they were driven backwards and forwards from one trouble to the other, until they had discovered a mean distance at which they could most tolerably exist.

Schopenhauer, *Parerga and Paralipomena*

The difficulties that obtain in any kind of professional organization, where intense individualization operates against co-operation, have been greatly multiplied in chiropractic. Its exponents have been hard to lead and as addicted to dispute as were the first few, who fought at every fleck and flicker in the chiropractic kaleidoscope. Continually working with the hands tends to make a man or woman self-sufficient, persecution breeds independence, and so nothing short of an extreme abiding danger common to all would have called those professionals to the colors and imbued them with an organization spirit.

Chittenden Turner, *The Rise of Chiropractic*

FATHER AND SON

On October 20, 1913, D.D. Palmer died at his home on West Vernon Avenue in Los Angeles, the victim of typhoid fever complicated by a "tendency for years to brain congestion." Even his passing, however, could not end longstanding animosities between Palmer (fig. 1) and his son Bartlett Joshua (B.J.), the heir and self-styled Developer of chiropractic

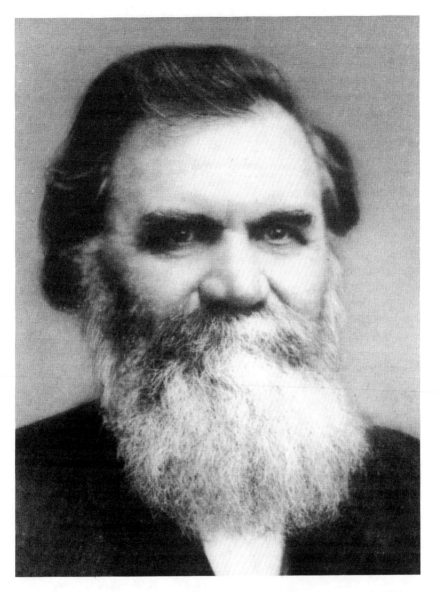

FIGURE 1. Daniel David (D.D.) Palmer. From *B.J. Palmer Chiropractic Clinic Pictorial*, c. 1950. Courtesy of David D. Palmer Health Sciences Library.

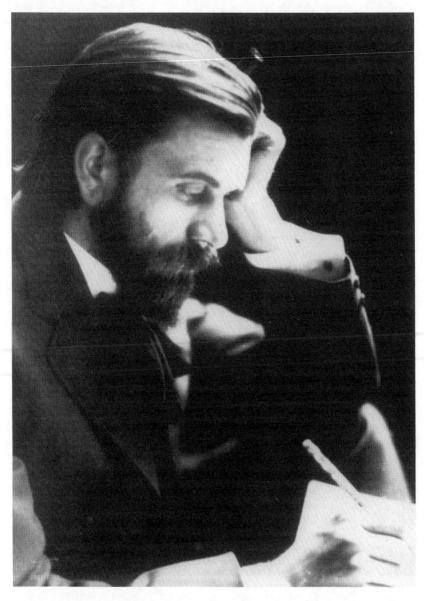

FIGURE 2. Bartlett Joshua (B.J.) Palmer. Courtesy of David D. Palmer Health
Sciences Library.

(fig. 2). Joy M. Loban, executor of D.D.'s estate and head of B.J.'s rival Universal Chiropractic College, filed suit alleging that B.J. had maliciously and intentionally struck his father with an automobile during a lyceum parade at the Palmer School in August 1913, resulting in injuries that caused D.D.'s death.[1]

But supporting evidence was scant. The elder Palmer was visiting friends in the Davenport area during the summer of 1913[2] and had accepted an invitation from B.J. to participate in the procession down Brady Street. Assigned to ride alone in the lead car behind an American flag and marching band, D.D. became eager for the affair to begin. He bolted from the automobile, moved toward the flag, and motioned the band to march. Confusion followed. B.J., driving the second car in the review, steered out of line and moved near to where D.D. stood. Entreaties for D.D. to enter the car failed. D.D. ran across the road and then three blocks down Brady Street until he stopped beside officials of the Universal Chiropractic College. As the parade approached, he jumped into the street and led the march for a block until police officers escorted him from the procession. Apparently uninjured, Palmer prepared to leave the next day for his California home.[3]

The suit filed in the wake of D.D.'s death seemed to be a ploy on the part of Loban and the Universal College to discredit B.J. and to disrupt the operations of the Palmer School. The charges became a rallying cry for chiropractic dissidents who opposed the younger Palmer. After winding through the courts for several months, the case was dismissed in December 1914 by a grand jury who threatened to investigate the motives of the instigators.[4] Alongside his defenders, D.D. Palmer's contentious spirit seemed to be bickering with his son even from the grave. The affair itself serves as an appropriate symbol for the schismatic and turbulent nature of chiropractic itself.

The parade incident was the fruit of continuing enmity between father and son which had produced the original chiropractic rift years before. Barely thirteen at the time of the first adjustment in September 1895, B.J. became absorbed in his father's emerging ideas and techniques, assisting him in spinal manipulations on a variety of cases. Initially, the elder Palmer wanted to retain chiropractic as a family secret and conducted his cures in darkened rooms with drawn drapes, fearful that his discovery would be stolen. B.J. began arguing that chiropractic should be taught beyond the family circle, extending the benefits (and the prestige of the Palmers) to a wider world. A narrow escape from a railway accident in Clinton Junction, Illinois, in late 1897 made the senior Palmer acutely aware that his innovation would be snuffed out if he died and helped convince him to teach the new system at the Palmer School and Cure.[5]

This relatively minor row between father and son soon intensified as the school drew few to its erratic course of informal and tutorial instruction. An 1899 graduate explained that with his $500 tuition came "no blackboards, no text books, no notes, not a single lecture. For six days I witnessed the giving of a number of treatments. That was the sum total of information that was transferred in exchange for the tuition paid."[6] By January 1902, only fifteen students had graduated. Late that year and without explanation, D.D. Palmer suddenly packed his belongings (including all of the bedding from the school infirmary) and moved to Portland, Oregon, apparently disheartened by sluggish school growth, an $8,000 debt, and potential legal troubles. B.J., barely twenty years old and himself a 1902 graduate, assumed control of the spare facility by default, mollified insistent creditors, and gradually pulled the school from debt. In Portland, D.D. taught chiropractic to two medical doctors, and together they opened the Portland College of Chiropractic. Within a year, however, his partners dismissed him from the school and Palmer traveled the West Coast giving chiropractic demonstrations. He returned to Davenport sometime in 1904 and established an uneasy, equal partnership with the now confident and flamboyant son who had kept the school afloat in his absence.[7]

D.D. Palmer attempted to regain his preeminence but soon became enmeshed in legal troubles. On October 7, 1905, he was indicted for practicing medicine without a license and after two continuances was tried on March 27, 1906, in a Scott County, Iowa, courtroom. In a brief two-day trial, the jury found him guilty and District Court Judge A.P. Barker gave him a choice between 105 days in the county jail and a $350 fine. Palmer chose the jail term and sought to use *The Davenport Democrat and Leader* as a platform for denouncing his persecution and for lauding chiropractic. He also believed that refusing to pay his fine created an unwelcome financial burden on the state in both court costs and jail expenses and that, if other prosecuted chiropractors followed his example, future legal action against the profession would be minimized.[8] But weariness and the restrictions of a nine- by eleven-foot cell soon overcame principle. After serving only twenty-three days, Palmer paid the full fine plus $39.50 in court costs and walked free.[9]

After his release, Palmer returned to the school and sought entry. B.J. met his father at the door and refused him access to the building or grounds, advising him that he no longer held property interests in the school. Technically, B.J. was right. Only a few days before, upon the advice of attorney Willard Carver, D.D. had transferred his property rights to Mabel Palmer, B.J.'s wife, to forestall future legal difficulties. The two Palmers were unable to resolve the ensuing feud over control of school property and submitted their squabble to a committee of arbitration. On May 1, 1906, D.D. Palmer accepted $2,196.79 from his son in payment for his interests. Bitter and distraught from the rift, the elder Palmer moved to the Indian Territory of Medford, Oklahoma (where his brother published a local newspaper), and temporarily took up a grocery and goldfish business before reestablishing a chiropractic career.[10]

D.D. Palmer remained bitter for the rest of his life over his ouster from the Davenport school. He claimed that the "boy chiro" B.J. was a "sneak-thief" and a "rascal" who robbed his "parental benefactor" of due honor and stole chiropractic away. But this first chiropractic schism ran deeper than personal animosity. D.D. believed that his son was a dilettante, guilty of bastardizing basic chiropractic concepts and teaching ignorance compounded by youthful exuberance. According to the senior Palmer, B.J.'s notion that all nerves originated in the brain and passed energy down the spinal cord through the intervertebral foramina to the various parts of the body by "direct mental impulse" was anatomical nonsense that denied the existence of spinal or sympathetic nerves and threatened to turn chiropractic into a laughingstock. From D.D.'s perspective, physiological short-cuts such as this "direct nerve system" were features of his son's misunderstanding of Innate Intelligence, the operation of Universal Spirit through individual Matter. B.J. held that Innate Intelligence in each being resided next to (and presumably empowered) the brain, which passed impulses through nerves by direct mechanical action. The body acted as a machine driven by the brain. The brain therefore took preeminence in governing bodily operation, consigning Universal Intelligence to a secondary role, allowing God simply "the opportunity to express its quantities through man." D.D. objected vehemently to the man-as-machine metaphor and to the limited and ambiguous role granted to both Universal and Innate Intelligence. According to the founder of chiropractic, B.J. was incapable of offering an intelligent explanation of Innate.[11]

D.D.'s criticism was disingenuous. These objections reflected his most developed position on Universal and Innate Intelligence as expressed in *The Science, Art and Philosophy of Chiropractic,* published in 1910. In "The Chiropractic," an 1899 pamphlet, he had himself described human beings as "human machines" that would run smoothly if all parts were in their proper places, a notion undoubtedly taught to the younger Palmer. In the pamphlet D.D. had also mentioned ill-defined "vital fluids and forces" reminiscent of the harmonialism of magnetic healing, but the machine imagery dominated.[12] This early mechanistic position in his chiropractic career may have been an attempt to escape the metaphysical side of magnetic healing that earlier had made him a target for the quack label; the man-as-machine concept seemed more scientific in a machine age. In light of D.D.'s entire career, however, this machine metaphor is the aberration. In 1904 he tentatively unveiled Innate Intelligence to the profession,[13] and in February 1906 "Immortality" appeared in *The Chiroprac-*

tor, presenting in abridged form the concepts of Universal, Innate, and Educated Intelligence that were developed more extensively in his 1910 tome. After a brief flirtation with a mechanistic position, D.D. had clearly rejected the idea as inadequate and once again embraced the familiar harmonial notions associated with magnetic healing, now updated for chiropractic.[14]

By 1910, D.D. was ready to censure his son for adopting "brain power" as the unseen life force and for the body-as-machine idea he had come to abhor. The young B.J. had probably been confused in trying to sort through the jumble of mechanistic and harmonial teachings presented in his father's idiosyncratic language. How then had the young B.J., a high school dropout with little formal education, moved from these early, often muddled ideas of his father to the "philosophy" that the brain was the power source of the body and come to promote himself as the "philosophical counsel" and polestar of the profession? A chiropractic trial in Wisconsin had spurred the transformation.

In 1907, Japanese chiropractor and recent Palmer graduate Shegataro Morikubo was charged in La Crosse, Wisconsin, with illegally practicing medicine, surgery, and osteopathy. B.J. traveled to his aid and hired defense attorney Tom Morris, a well-known local figure then serving as a state legislator in the camp of Progressive Governor Robert LaFollette. Morris had just two weeks to prepare for the August 13 trial, with only the failure of D.D. Palmer in Iowa the previous year as a precedent for countering similar charges. During his preparation Morris discovered *Modernized Chiropractic,* the profession's first textbook, published in 1906 by Solon Langworthy, Oakley Smith, and Minora Paxson, three early disciples of D.D. who had severed ties with Davenport and launched the rival American School of Chiropractic and Nature Cure in Cedar Rapids, Iowa. *Modernized Chiropractic* provided Morris with a distinction between chiropractic and osteopathy in philosophy as well as technique, describing the brain and not the blood (as osteopaths maintained) as the unseen fountain of power for the body and detailing the "chiropractic thrust" as distinct from other spinal techniques. Cleverly, Morris had the charge amended to practicing osteopathy without a license and, by drawing on Langworthy's book, proceeded to demonstrate that chiropractic differed from osteopathy and from other sciences because of dissimilarities in manipulative technique *and* differences in philosophy. The jury deliberated less than a half hour and acquitted Morikubo. In the wake of this success, B.J. appropriated the concepts of *Modernized Chiropractic* as interpreted by Tom Morris and wrote frequently of brain power and chiropractic "philosophy" in terms sounding suspiciously like those he had heard in the courtroom.[15]

The result was confusion in chiropractic ranks over the meaning of "philosophy" for the profession. B.J. began mixing what was actually a medical philosophy in *Modernized Chiropractic* with the harmonial philosophy of his father. But B.J.'s brand of chiropractic philosophy was confined increasingly to speculations on Matter rather than Spirit, a philosophy of *practice* showcasing medical and scientific theories for which he had no solid proof rather than esoteric notions of Universal and Innate Intelligence. B.J., by late 1907 the self-styled "Developer" of chiropractic, was business-minded and, in operating the "Fountainhead" Palmer school, came to emphasize the spine instead of the cosmos. The harmonial ideas remained important for gaining converts to the chiropractic cause but evolved into a hardened orthodoxy, a backdrop for the more immediately relevant and practical task of adjusting patients and relieving pain. A perfunctory invocation of Innate along with B.J.'s "philosophy" of practice (including whatever medical ideas and adjustment techniques he might promote) became the fundamentals of the chiropractic faith, the test of orthodoxy for those who wanted to practice "S. P. & U." (specific, pure, and unadulterated) or "straight" chiropractic. B.J. condemned dissenters or "mixers" as "medipractors" and "chiropracTOIDS" and in turn was denounced variously as the "Medical Mussolini," the "Mad Mullah" and "Tsar of Chiropractic," the "bewhiskered Janus of Davenport."[16]

Since B.J. Palmer and his colleagues coined the terms "straights" and "mixers," most chiropractors have followed their lead, reducing the schism in their ranks to this dichotomy. The straights are taken to be those who adhere strictly to the original principles of Palmer chiropractic, locating the cause of disease at the spine and providing relief by adjusting the spinal column only. The "mixers" were those chiropractic apostates who abandoned the initial precepts (which often became whatever the straights claimed them to be) and developed a host of "new moves" and adjunct modalities to treat their patients.[17] Adherence to this dichotomy, however, focuses on technique and has obscured both differences between father and son and a more complex evolution in the chiropractic schism.

HARMONISTS AND MECHANICS

The most fundamental division in the development of chiropractic is between those advocates who approach health in the spiritual, harmonial tradition and those who follow the mechanical path. On a more modest scale, this chiropractic split replicates the conflict evident more than three centuries before at the dawn of the scientific revolution. Harmonial chiropractors in the style of D.D. Palmer viewed themselves as champions of Life, high scientists endowed with the gnosis of health who understood the movement of Spirit within Matter. Many chiropractors, however, while applauding the merits of natural, drugless techniques, became unsettled by the cultist atmosphere and sought scientific respectability by culling from chiropractic a more rational approach, appropriating the values of the mechanical tradition that informed the orthodox medical marketplace of the early twentieth century. The schism kept chiropractic in constant inner turmoil, but the division provided a place within the profession for practitioners of varied temperaments. The derision of orthodox medicine kept most of the mechanical rationalists within ranks, pushing chiropractors toward a measure of cohesion they were often unable to achieve by themselves.

Viewing the basic chiropractic schism as a rift between harmonists and mechanics, rather than simply between straights and mixers, allows a more accurate description of chiropractic development. D.D. Palmer stands as the harmonial straight, combining the philosophy and vital power of Innate with the hand adjustment of subluxated vertebrae as the only method of curing disease. B.J. became the quasi-harmonial straight, invoking Innate but focusing on *medical* philosophy and the techniques of spinal adjustment. While continuing to bicker between themselves, both the Founder and the Developer were quick to condemn anyone who "mixed" other methods under the guise of chiropractic. In the process, they failed to recognize that a harmonial approach was possible even for a mixer.

The quintessential early mixer as denounced by the Palmers was Willard Carver, D.D. Palmer's attorney who had advised him in the 1906 jail cell to transfer his property rights in the Palmer school to B.J.'s wife as protection against future legal action. As a boy Carver, born in Maysville, Iowa, in July 1866, had delivered chickens to D.D.'s grocery store in What Cheer, and Carver remained a long-time friend of the family. His mother Eliza, known affectionately as "slickhead" because of her straight-back hairstyle and her shrewdness,[18] became one of D.D.'s first patients when Palmer turned to healing. Even though Carver received a degree from Drake University and began practicing law, he took an ardent interest in the relationship between psychology and health, eventually fashioning a system he called Relatolity. At first he was satisfied to serve as legal counsel to struggling chiropractors, but soon he decided to become directly involved and infuse the movement with his own developing notions of health and disease. In June 1906 he graduated from the Charles Ray Parker School of Chiropractic in Ottumwa and with a business partner established his own institute in Oklahoma City, the Carver-Denny School, chartered in 1908 as the Carver Chiropractic College. Not to be outdone by the Palmers, he styled himself the "Constructor" of chiropractic and dubbed his school the "Science Head" in contrast to the "Fountainhead" Palmer school in Davenport.[19]

Carver developed a harmonial approach similar to D.D. Palmer's own eventual synthesis, but the two argued frequently over the science and philosophy behind chiropractic. Carver was a mixer as the Palmers charged, but a harmonial one not as far out of step as they imagined. At odds with the straights, Carver held that nerve interference can occur in areas of the body other than the spine, emulating the osteopathic approach, which designated manipulation at bodily joints and structures other than the vertebrae. B.J. especially condemned Carver for his "structural" analysis, a mechanical engineering concept that viewed the spinal column as a weight-bearing unit adapting to gravity. In this view, areas of potential weakness and failure could be determined through close, scientific examination. In contrast, the Palmers advanced the "bone-out-of-place" or "segmental" theory, that isolated vertebrae become misaligned autonomously. Subluxation theory remained for years a major source of contention between Carver and the younger Palmer and between mixers and straights.[20]

Carver also advocated suggestion as a major therapeutic adjunct to the actual manipulation. In a letter on February 15, 1905, at a time when D.D. Palmer was still developing the function of Innate in the world, Carver wrote to the Palmers explaining that chiropractic and suggestion were both sciences identical in object and application, "inseparable twins" that could not be divorced successfully from practice. According to Carver, suggestion was not a treatment of disease per se but corrected the cause of bodily ills stemming from the subjective mind (such as a tobacco habit or insanity), those ailments not created by a mechanical problem in the human structure. Chiropractic is limited to the mechanical while suggestion, argued Carver, "*goes back* further than the mechanical, to the very foundation of life, and has to do with an intelligence which existed before there was a bony structure to luxate." Carver begged the Palmers "not to maim a universal law of cure" by separating it and embracing only the smaller part. "It is because I love Chiro as ardently as a schoolboy his first sweetheart," Carver ended, "that I beg of you to bring the science of suggestion down to date and make it the working companion of adjustment."[21]

For Carver, Palmer chiropractic was limited to the mechanical and needed completion by adding suggestion to its therapeutic arsenal, an adjunct that would then give chiropractic a true claim to high science. D.D. Palmer considered Carver's idea worthy of consideration but by 1910 was ready to announce confidently to Carver and the world that "all diseased conditions," including mental aberrations, resulted from bone luxations and could be cured only by mechanical adjustment. For example, Palmer claimed to have cured a Dr. Story of insanity by replacing his fourth cervical vertebra after treatment by "a very prominent healer who used Suggestive Therapeutics" had failed.[22] Palmer believed that *his* chiropractic already contained a complete view of life, that the mechanical adjustment of the spine was the *only* thing that kept Innate from achieving full fruition in the world. Suggestion then, in Palmer's view, unnecessarily complicated an already simple and true system; Carver threatened to invest chiropractic with a complexity that Palmer had escaped.

By the time of the Founder's public censure, Carver had staked a considerable claim on the fortunes of chiropractic through the operation of his Oklahoma school. He stayed loosely within the ranks of chiropractic but incorporated the views on suggestion rejected by the Palmers into the "Science of Relatolity," his own harmonial "Science of the Soul." In June 1913, he began a series of public lectures at Carver College detailing the "peerless leaders of all system[s]." The application of his principles, he promised, was destined for adoption by all countries of the world and would usher in a millennium of health, "the eventual evolution of human beings, to such perfection, as to eliminate abnormality, except as the result of occasional trauma." His views, however, echoed the major themes of D.D. Palmer, who was never mentioned. Carver defined the Soul as the "non-material, Intelligent Life Power," the "Indestructible Life" imminent in humans and causing all animation, the power Palmer had called Innate Intelligence. In addition to the Soul, the individual possesses "Consciousness," a entity similar to Palmer's Educated Intelligence. The Soul produces Consciousness and is ever-willing to impart the "Immaculate Intelligence" from the "Great Soul of the Universe" through "impressions" to the Consciousness, which then translates them into thought and language. Consciousness is the earth-bound receptacle of intelligence from Soul, but in turn Consciousness must transmit information from the physical environment through its five senses back to the Soul. Without the eyes and ears of Consciousness, the Soul "would never be advised of man's physical existence, for the Soul would have no avenue through which it could receive that fact." Consciousness is the comprehensive term describing the material intelligence of man; Soul encompasses his psychic intelligence. Together, Carver held, these two phases completely explain human intelligence.[23]

D.D. Palmer would have no basic qualm with this position. What he objected to was Carver's inclusion of suggestion, an addition that Carver developed more fully in his lecture series. In the "psychologic phase," Consciousness transmits a suggestion to the Soul in such a way that it is "evolved into cognizance." In the "biological phase," the material being transmits intelligence to the Soul and the Soul then operates on the suggestion by conveying power through the nerve system to all parts of the body. In practical terms, the suggestion creates an actual physiological response in the nervous system and is a commonplace experience. The cells of the body constantly transmit information to the Soul (which passes through the brain with or without producing consciousness of it), and the Consciousness of the individual actively transmits data to the Soul by autosuggestion. Through signs, tokens, pictures, and written and spoken language, the Consciousness of one individual also imparts intelligence to the Consciousness of another. But this ordinary means of suggestion from one individual to another is constricted by the medium of the senses. Telepathy, whether volitional or involitional, overcomes this constraint, providing an extrasensual mode of suggestion. Doctors who develop telepathic rapport can receive information from the diseased bodies of their patients which offer guidance for treatment. Suggestion itself, whether spoken or telepathic, can succeed only if the physical avenue of the body is in harmony, allowing unobstructed transmission of intelligence first to the Soul and then from the Soul to every part of the body. The disharmony or "disrelationship" of bodily structures prohibits the flow of intelligence through the brain and nerves. Before suggestion can be effective, the therapist must apply "extraneous physical aid," a manual manipulation that restores structural harmony. Before restoration, "Kenetic-Soul-Power" was destructive to the body because it was deflected from traveling through its constructive nerve channels; after restoration it resumes a proper harmonious flow. According to Carver, Christian Science and other psychologies failed to recognize that disharmony in the physical structure impeded the effects of suggestion, an incomplete view that his science corrected. Carver's Relatolity, the "Science of Relationship," combined Suggestive Therapeutics with manipulation, offering the therapist a comprehensive, harmonial world view and a drugless armamentarium for mastering the ills of mankind.[24]

Unlike Carver, other early chiropractors ignored the philosophical component of D.D. Palmer's thought and focused on the mechanical adjustment, founding schools and developing techniques at odds with Palmer's. Whereas the harmonial chiropractors offered plenary truth, the spine doctors within the movement sought to move chiropractic away from sectarian dogma and into the medical mainstream by offering particular truth, the expertise of the specialist. Lyndon Lee, a New York chiropractor, expressed this more limited view clearly.

> Employing a doctor should be no different from buying any other commodity of a daily need. The healing professions as a whole can be considered a store in which various brands of health service are for sale. When illness overtakes us we enter this store seeking the department in which is sold the particular service suited to our requirements. There is the department of Chiropractic, Allopathy, homeopathy and of osteopathy. In each department are specialists to cater to our wants. They listen to the description of our condition and, like salesmen, recommend such of their wares as they feel will meet our situation.[25]

A number of D.D. Palmer's earliest followers abandoned the spiritual overtones then in embryonic form and began developing chiropractic as a spinal speciality soon after taking the Palmer course. Probably the most important for the survival of chiropractic was Solon M. Langworthy (born 1868), a 1901 graduate, who also received a diploma that same year from a school in Kansas City, Missouri, called the American College of Manual Therapeutics.[26] Langworthy opened an office in Cedar Rapids, Iowa, in July 1901 and soon developed an infirmary known as the "Health Home." By 1903 he had launched the American School of Chiropractic and Nature Cure, training new chiropractors at a time when D.D. Palmer had fled to Portland, Oregon, leaving the Palmer school to a stripling B.J. and chiropractic to an uncertain future. Langworthy attempted to cast chiropractic as a science in the mechanical tradition, concerned solely with Matter and acceptable to twentieth-century researchers. In October 1903, he began publishing *Backbone,* a chiropractic journal whose title indicated his chief focus, styling it to approach the subject with a dignity that the broadsides and testimonial copy of the Palmers and other irregular practitioners of the day failed to achieve. His physiological hypotheses linking the pathology of aging with the progressive compression of spinal discs and narrowing of the "spinal windows" or intervertebral foramina gained notice in the popular press, and in 1904 the Chicago *American* invited him to discuss his theories. *Modernized Chiropractic* (1906), the two-volume treatise Langworthy produced with 1899 Palmer graduates Minora C. Paxson and Oakley G. Smith, who had joined him in Cedar Rapids, consolidated his research and presented chiropractic with a scientific facelift.[27]

Langworthy evolved gradually from being a mechanical "straight," describing chiropractic as the rational science of "hand-fixing" only, to become a mechanical "mixer," employing a host of mechanical appliances which drew the particular ire of the Palmers. The "Amplia-Thrill" (fig. 3A), a patented traction table constructed to relieve compression, and the "Anatomical Adjuster," designed to stretch the spine, became important therapeutic adjuncts for his newly created "Spinal Extension Department" at the American School. In July 1904, Langworthy implemented a more rigorous curriculum, extending his course to two years (four five-month terms) at a time when the entire Palmer course lasted four months or less and including subjects foreign to the Palmer school, such as chemical diagnosis, urinalysis, histology, and microscopy. Armed with a respectable curriculum, Langworthy stood ready to back a chiropractic licensing bill in Minnesota, the first such law in the nation. In early 1905 a Langworthy associate maneuvered a bill through the Minnesota legislature which required a state board examination in courses similar to the Langworthy offerings and specified two years of training at an approved chiropractic school, mandates that the Palmer school could not match. D.D. Palmer made a fast trip to Minnesota's Governor Johnson, explained that the bill

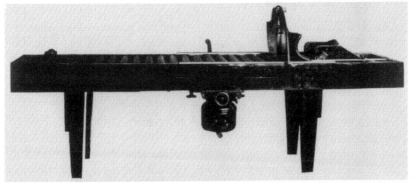

A

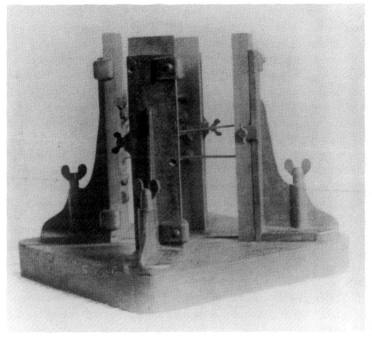

B

FIGURE 3. The Langworthy Amplia-Thrill (*A*) was described in 1932 as an "apparatus which by fixed traction creates negative pressure in the vertebral joints and by rapid non-violent intermittent traction produces spontaneity in the dormant cells surrounding the joints thereby reducing vertical subluxations by causing the intervertebral cartilages to increase in thickness." Smith's Situmounter (*B*) was described as a "device for mounting vertebral sections so that when cleaned they can be studied in the exact position which they held in the body at death." From Oakley Smith, *Naprapathic Genetics (Modernized Chiropractic)*, 2 vols. (Chicago, 1932), 1:275, 2:175.

embraced a definition of chiropractic beyond the scope of his discovery, and urged a prompt veto. With medical opposition to the bill also probably heavy, the governor vetoed the measure, arguing that chiropractic was as yet untried and unscientific. Palmer thus helped to scuttle the bill promoted by his "mixing" nemesis, a bill that would have given chiropractic official recognition for the first time.[28]

In addition to his squabbles with Langworthy, D.D. Palmer clashed with Langworthy associate Oakley Smith (1880–1967), another early disciple turned dissenter. Smith was dean of the faculty and vice-president at the American School until 1907, when he left Cedar Rapids to develop his own health discovery and organize his own school, the Chicago College of Naprapathy. In the early years of the decade, Smith had traveled to Czechoslovakia and was fascinated by the Bohemian peasant practice of napravit, a method of back massage for treating disease. His chiropractic background along with an avid interest in dissection spurred him to examine the physiological basis of the Bohemian system while at the American School. His "Situmounter" (fig. 3B), a precision instrument he invented for examining joint motion in spinal sections taken from cadavers, convinced him that the subluxation theory was wrong. The revelation was a great blow and set him on a quest for the principal cause of disease. Working at his microscope on November 16, 1905, Smith made his self-proclaimed "immortal discovery" at 8:45 P.M. that a "ligatite" (tight ligament) occurring near a nerve creates mechanical tension obstructing proper nerve flow, thereby causing numerous diseases. Repetitive, manual massage of the altered connective tissue, modeled after the Bohemian thrust, defined the distinctive naprapathic treatment or "stretchment." It was, according to Smith, a "miracle" health cure spawning a new science.[29]

Others who took the Palmer course would also shun the spiritual components and focus on Matter to discover their own miracle cures. Andrew P. Davis (1835–1915), an apprentice-trained M.D. and osteopathic physician who also dabbled in homeopathy, ophthalmology, otology, and orificial surgery, added the D.C. diploma from Palmer's School and Cure in 1898. In 1909, Davis published *Neuropathy,* detailing a novel combination uniting "three of the greatest modern sciences," osteopathy, chiropractic, and ophthalmology. Davis embraced the "best of every scientific, rational, natural method of cure for human ills ever presented to the human family," and his book suggested "every known means to remove causes of conditions called disease." Davis moved into the school business with his American School of Neuropathy, turning out neuropaths to spread the system. D.D. Palmer was unimpressed with Davis' medical "medley," ridiculing it as a "miserable subterfuge," a "pick up of anything and everything," a "mongrel of so many breeds that it would be impossible to get a correct pedigree."[30]

Conflict over the meaning of modern science brought continual disruption to the profession. J.F. Alan Howard, a disgruntled Palmer faculty member, organized the National School of Chiropractic in 1906 as a Davenport rival to the Palmer school after B.J. Palmer rejected his entreaties to emphasize research through human dissection. In 1908, Howard moved his institution to Chicago, where his students soon gained admittance to the clinics and autopsies of the Cook County Hospital, and hired William C. Schulze, a graduate of Rush Medical College, for his faculty, along with several additional doctors of medicine. National developed as the preeminent "mixer" school, broadening the scope of chiropractic to embrace the scientific method and rejecting the philosophy of Innate. "Our aim," National catalogs proclaimed as a gibe at the Palmer brand of chiropractic, "is toward rationalism, not radicalism."[31]

SALVATION FOR MIXERS: THE LYCEUM AS CAMP MEETING

By the time of the Founder's death in 1913, the chiropractic world was clearly in disarray, rife with schismatics and defectors. The graduates of D.D. Palmer had exhibited little sense of unity in hatching numerous varieties of chiropractic. B.J. Palmer, assuming the full mantle of leadership, sought to remold this divided world into a loyal band of chiropractors committed to the ideals of "pure and unadulterated" chiropractic as he defined them, weaned from the tentacles of the "Medical Octopus."[32] The Palmer School became the foundation for instilling evangelical fervor in his students. Harry Runge, an early disciple of the younger Palmer and a pioneer chiropractor in Massachusetts, explained that

> B.J. had the students so they could hardly wait until they could get out into practice, to carry chiropractic to the world, and to get sick people well. He filled us with enthusiasm and self-confidence. We knew that we had the power to do these things right in the palms of our hands. We were 'miracle men' . . . I wanted to be a pioneer, a leader, a martyr if necessary. I wanted to be B.J.'s representative in Boston.[33]

B.J. cultivated and revitalized this passion by inventing the annual chiropractic lyceum, a protracted, chiropractic camp meeting designed to uplift the faithful and to bring mixing dissenters back into the fold.

"Chiropractors From All the World Will Be Present at This Great Gathering" announced an advertisement in the *Davenport Democrat and Leader* for the first lyceum at the Fountainhead Palmer School, August 17–21, 1914.[34] Under the searing heat of a late-summer Iowa sun, B.J. combined hoopla, showmanship, and fervent oratory to inflame participants with a missionary zeal for his brand of straight chiropractic. By 1916, the lyceum attracted 3,064 registrants. Through the years an intriguing mix of name speakers such as Clarence Darrow, William Jennings Bryan, Elbert Hubbard, Bernarr Macfadden, Jascha Heifetz, James Corbett, and Bob Fitzsimmons added star appeal to the gathering.[35] Bombastic parades swarming through the streets of Davenport became another regular feature. As a centerpiece for these spectacles, B.J. constructed a huge, papier-mâché vertebrae. Marchers hoisted the segments on their shoulders and carried metal signs on their hips, each with a letter that together spelled "Chiropractic Fountainhead," a total of twenty-four letters, exactly the number of vertebrae in the spine.[36]

By 1921, the lyceum lasted a full week, complete with 8,000 chiropractors from around the globe, four miles of parades, and a huge picture of B.J. prominently displayed in downtown Davenport. With an eye toward practical pageantry, B.J. captured the gala on 5,000 feet of film and offered it for $25.00 per showing—"A GREAT BUSINESS PULLER" his rental ad promised.[37] These were heady times for the Palmer School, known throughout the profession as simply the PSC. A new administration building, clinic, and classrooms had been added to accommodate a steadily increasing flow of students and patients. By 1922, the PSC boasted 2,300 students representing every state and more than two dozen foreign countries and B.J. was broadcasting the "Wonders of Chiropractic" over WOC, the nation's second radio station. (In 1932, Ronald Reagan went to work for B.J., broadcasting from high atop the Chiropractic Fountainhead in Davenport, where, as Reagan signed off his shows, "the West begins and in the state where the tall corn grows").[38] B.J. was riding the crest of chiropractic; his school dominated the field.

The lyceum of 1923 initiated a dramatic decline in B.J.'s status and the fortunes of the PSC when he officially introduced the Neurocalometer, or NCM, a device that reputedly detected subluxations directly by determining changes in nerve transmission along the spine (fig. 4). Dossa D. Evins, a onetime electrical engineer, developed the NCM between 1920 and 1922 while taking the Palmer course and offered it to B.J. Traditionally, chiropractors sensed the location of a subluxation by hand palpation of the spine, searching for the "hot box" or spot of elevated surface heat which indicated the problem vertebra. The NCM, basically a galvanometer or thermocouple millivoltmeter, was designed to register the phenomenon, removing imprecision and guesswork from the examination. B.J. promised that it would convert chiropractors from "dogmatists" to "human scientists."[39] Straight chiropractors, who had hailed B.J. as a virtual demigod, were bewildered by his attempt to revolutionize chiropractic through such a device. In addition, his marketing strategy struck many as greedy, grasping commercialism. B.J. devised a leasing plan for the Neurocalometer which seems to have been modeled after Albert Abrams's distribution of the

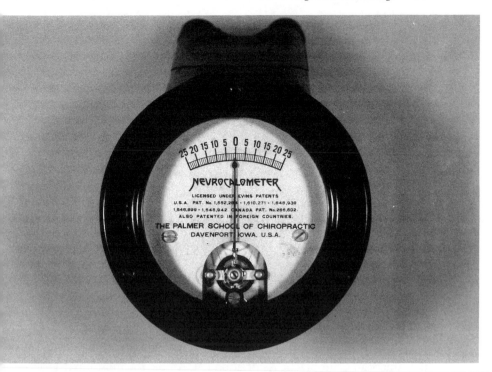

FIGURE 4. The Neurocalometer. Courtesy of Logan College of Chiropractic Archives, Chesterfield, Missouri.

famous "Oscilloclast." This electrical gadget, endorsed by Upton Sinclair, purported to cure disease by producing vibrations that would correct abnormal organ oscillations first diagnosed through ERA, the "electronic reactions of Abrams."[40] The Neurocalometer, like the Oscilloclast, could not be purchased outright. Chiropractors leased the NCM for a lofty $2,000 on the installment plan, with an initial cash payment of $600. The contract required the lessee to charge his patients a minimum of ten dollars per reading or suffer possible forfeit. The deal included an inspection service providing semiannual visits from a traveling corps of Palmer-trained NCM technicians. Subscribers were to attend the 1924 Lyceum for instruction in proper technique.[41]

The months preceding the lyceum exploded in controversy. Fear of losing business to NCM-equipped chiropractors induced many to buy. Others who could not raise the down payment considered cheaper, knock-off versions from Palmer competitors graced with names such as Neuropyr-ometer, Neurothermometer, Neurophonometer, and the less elegantly named Hotbox Indicator. B.J. constantly threatened legal action against these "sycophants, bloodsuckers," and "spittle-lickers" from the pages of his *Fountain Head News,* even though the patents-applied-for status of the NCM left it in legal limbo.[42] In late August, scores of confused and concerned chiropractors huddled under the lyceum tent, waiting expectantly for the word from Davenport.

B.J. responded with "The Hour Has Struck," a controversial speech that rocked the profession. The Neurocalometer, he proclaimed, will usher in a bright era with a new foundation for chiropractic. Spinal pressures that before were hidden from the chiropractor now stand revealed by the scientific instrument. Those who fail to employ the NCM will be forced from business, he assured them—only his device could indicate the place for adjustment. Chiropractic accomplishments of the past stand as worthless and insignificant when compared to the glorious future guaranteed by the revolutionary Neurocalometer. The NCM is the redeemer of the profession; the hour has struck, B.J. declared, for separating the chiropractic "milkers" from the "feeders."[43]

Chiropractors around the country were stunned by B.J.'s address. Many saw it as a naked ploy for making money and for coercing allegiance to the Palmer brand of chiropractic. Only members of the Universal Chiropractors Association (UCA), B.J.'s organization of straight chiropractors started in 1906, could lease a Neurocalometer. Those who belonged to the American Chiropractic Association (ACA), the foremost mixer group formed in 1922, or held any affiliation hostile to the UCA were barred from leasing.[44] These restrictions along with the exorbitant price of the device infuriated many state societies already at odds with the UCA. The Hoosier Chiropractors' Association printed a resolution in its *Central States Bulletin* condemning B.J. for his attempt "to intimidate chiropractors, to hold a monopoly upon the chiropractic profession, and to increase his own personal fortune by perhaps two millions of dollars." "The issue is clear cut," the editor continued. "Palmer has made the division, it is Palmer and one thousand chiropractors against the field. Every chiropractor must take his stand and choose his side."[45] Lyndon Lee, aligned with the ACA as president of the New York State Chiropractic Society, prepared to offer his state members an NCM look-alike with identical parts manufactured by the same company that produced the NCM. Members would lease the machine for $200 down and $2.00 per month rental. The rental fee would substitute for dues to the society, and those who were delinquent could have the instrument recalled. Nonmembers could also lease—for $250 down and $5.00 monthly—a coercion of the pocketbook making membership in the organization quite attractive.[46]

The revolt against B.J. was not confined to the organizational schism already in place. Students and faculty at the PSC also split over the controversy. Some three-fourths of the school left, many retaining personal loyalty to B.J. but upset over the distribution of the Neurocalometer. In September 1926, disaffected Palmer faculty chairmen James N. Firth, Harry E. Vedder, Stephen J. Burich, and Arthur G. Hendricks, known as the "Big Four," opened the Lincoln Chiropractic College in Indianapolis, garnering a significant number of students.[47] Through the years the conflict between B.J. and the Big Four grew vehement, yet often amusing. In the "Fable of the Bed-Room Pottie That Became a Dignified 'Container,' or The Tale of The Urine That Went to College to Study 'Chiropractic,'" B.J. blasted the Lincoln College emphasis on urinalysis by graphically detailing the collection and voyage of a urine specimen mailed to the school. "What next 'chiropractic' college will go them one better by opening a urine AND SPUTUM endowment?" B.J. chided. "It appears that CHIROPRACTORS should sneak up on the low blind-belly-side, stick forth cute little 'containers,' gather sick refuse excrescences, bottle them, mail them to a 'chiropractic' college where they will be gazed upon when the urine is old." Reaction to the article was swift and impassioned. Earl C. Bailey, a chiropractor in New Bedford, Massachusetts, expressed a widespread view when he complained to B.J., protesting the piece in what he called B.J.'s "dearly beloved scandal sheet." "No fanatical leader of any age or any thought," Bailey wrote, "ever assumed the dictatorial power to shape the mind and actions of a group of followers as has B.J. Palmer." His sign-off provided a capsule review of his sentiments: "Yours for Chiropractic and Less Bunkum."[48]

Such outbursts clearly demonstrated that B.J.'s dominance in the profession slipped badly in the wake of the Neurocalometer debacle, but he continued to maintain his posture as chiropractic savior and used the lyceum to promise absolution to the wayward "mixing" brethren who would foresake their errors. In 1927, B.J. offered reconciliation, a perennial theme, at his "Back-to-the-Back Revival Lyceum," yet threatened a possible end to the era of grace.

> Be you anti-anything, or anti-everything, come and get one week of intensified B.J. so you can go home batteries recharged, bubbling over, brimming full of genuine CHIROPRACTIC shorn of everything medical.
>
> Be you the worst mixer in the world you are as welcome as the straightest laced we have.
>
> The spirit and intent of THIS lyceum will be to bring back into the fold all who have strayed and to make stronger those who have stayed in the fold.
>
> You may never get such a chance again. 'Nuf Sed![49]

But B.J. was preaching to the converted. Lyceum attendance was now measured in hundreds rather than thousands; the glory days of the pre-NCM lyceums had vanished. For thousands of chiropractors, B.J. had abused his authority and was no longer worthy of uncritical devotion. Many believed that he had forsaken pure chiropractic and prostituted himself with devices, profiting at the expense of the chiropractor in the field. With the NCM scheme, it appeared that B.J. had violated Aristotle's dictum of sage leadership: "A just ruler seems to make nothing out of his office; for he does not allot himself a larger share of things generally good, unless it be proportionate to his merits."[50]

THE DEVICE MANIA

From B.J.'s perspective, the use of devices per se was not heretical to the principles of pure chiropractic. The devices he sponsored, such as the X-ray in 1909 and the Neurocalometer in 1923, were designed not to treat the patient directly, but only to guide the chiropractor to the vertebrae requiring adjustment. This distinction, however, seemed to be lost on numerous chiropractors, and the Neurocalometer controversy intensified the movement toward mechanical devices or "modalities," whether intended to treat directly or merely assist. B.J. himself followed the trend at the 1936 lyceum by unveiling the Neurocalograph, an electric "graphometer" that recorded readings from the NCM. In the late thirties two more adjuncts appeared, his Neurotempometer, designed to hold the NCM and regulate its speed while passing down the patient's spine, and the grandiloquent, tongue-twisting Electroencephaloneuromentimpograph (fig. 5), which recorded "mental impulses sent out by Innate, over the fibers of the nervous system."[51]

The Neurocalometer and its companion devices opened the way for a Pandora's box of instruments that often beguiled the chiropractor. Straight, harmonial Palmerites were disheartened and confused by B.J.'s emphasis on machines; the definition of "pure" chiropractic was blurred. Some tried to recapture a fundamentalist, ultrastraight chiropractic by following D.D. Palmer's admonition that no electrical apparatus should find its way into an adjusting room,[52] while many with mixer tendencies moved toward pan-therapy, choosing from an array of "scientific" instruments parading before them. Determining the efficacy of any particular one became a daunting task. Chiropractors often fell as easy prey to device merchants who promised astonishing cures with miracle machines.

Some chiropractors became Chromo-Therapists by adopting the Chromaray, a device promoted by the Ernest Distributing Company of Milwaukee. This instrument used the "healing power of the Spectral Colors" as "nature's assistant" (fig. 6). E.A. Ernest based his instrument on a decades-old book, *The Principles of Light and Color* (1878) by Edwin D. Babbitt, the same Babbitt who had taught D.D. Palmer the techniques of

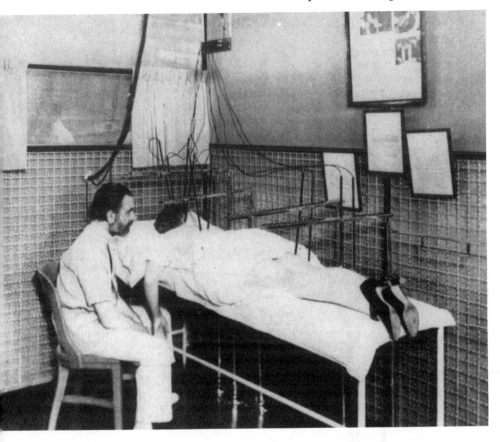

FIGURE 5. The Electroencephaloneuromentimpograph. (B.J. Palmer attending patient.) From *B.J. Palmer Chiropractic Clinic Pictorial*, c. 1950. Courtesy of David D. Palmer Health Sciences Library.

magnetic healing in the late nineteenth century through *Vital Magnetism: The Life Fountain.* Chromopathy was a harmonial-style therapy based on the notion that everything in the universe had its own particular color oscillation frequently undetected by the human eye, a type of visual counterpart to Albert Abrams's ERA theory that all substances are in a state of vibration. In a variation on the ancient doctrine of signatures, that an organ might be cured by an herb with the same shape or color—a heart-shaped plant would cure heart ailments, for example—chromopathy held that each color had its own peculiar power and was therapeutically effective against maladies of corresponding color. For example, the application of red rays through ruby glass would arouse the arterial blood; purple rays directed

CHROMARAY

The Scientific Way to Health with the
SEVEN COLORS of the SPECTRUM

Portable Combination Instrument

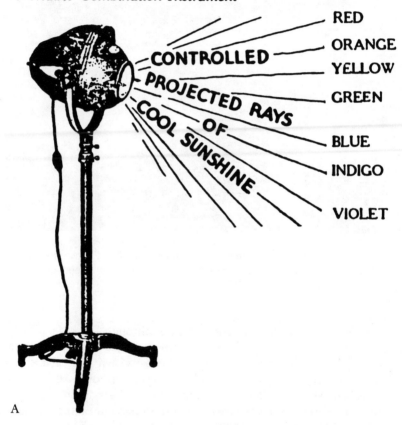

RED

ORANGE

YELLOW

GREEN

BLUE

INDIGO

VIOLET

A

FIGURE 6 (*A* and *B*). The Chromaray. From E. Ruscheweyh and E. A. Ernest, comps., *Operator's Manual* (Milwaukee: Ernest Distributing, 1937). Courtesy of Logan College of Chiropractic Archives, Chesterfield, Missouri.

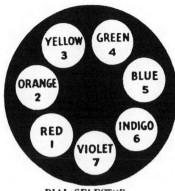

The colors in Chromaray are arranged numerically, eliminating confusion. Combinations are made by placing the desired number on the Sector A directly back of the desired number on the Dial Selector B, both appearing at the top in center of instrument. For instance, when combination No. 7+1 is specified, set the Dial Selector with Seven at top and the Sector with One at top.

B _____

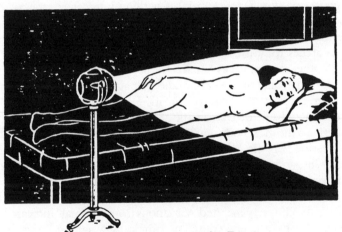

General Treatment on the Front

Chromaray-Focoray treatments afford complete relaxation for the patient and provide equal comfort in summer and winter. (No heat. No goggles required.)

It is applicable to both large and small areas (extended or restricted) for chronic or acute disorders.

Duration of Treatments

General (Front or Back)............................15 to 30 minutes.*
(Set instrument at angle about three feet from patient.)

Local ....15 to 30 minutes.
(Set instrument about 18 inches from patient, covering an area about 12 inches in diameter.)

Focorays (FO) with concentrated lens removed.............15 minutes.
(Set instrument about 12 inches from patient, covering area 2 to 3 inches in diameter.)

Focorays (FOC) with concentrated lens attached......5 to 15 minutes.
(Lens should be about 3 inches from patient, covering area ½ inch in diameter.)

Distance decreases intensity of color and increases area covered.

through purple glass would animate the venous blood and the digestive system. An intricate system of single colors and color combinations dialed on the Chromaray emitted "harnessed sunshine" and gave Chromo-Therapists a drugless treatment for most disorders, a "natural agent neutralizing the body through broken up Light." The chromopathist treated "causes" instead of "effects" and understood that integration of Mind and Soul with Body was necessary for health and harmony. Chromotherapy, noted the operator's manual, "is a tremendous step forward in the evolution of the Healing Science, not only because it makes use of the higher forces of nature, but because it works in accordance with the individuality of the patient instead of book theories and generalities." Results, therefore, were "amazing and permanent."[53]

Other chiropractors were lured instead by electricity and experimented with devices that had gained some currency within regular medicine. The McIntosh Electrical Corporation of Chicago offered the "Polysine" generator (fig. 7), an apparatus with an impressive array of special accessories which delivered low-voltage sinusoidal and galvanic currents for treating dozens of afflictions ranging from Bell's palsy to dysmenorrhea to fallen arches to goitre to "hiccough, persistent" to lumbago to "wrist drop."[54] Other chiropractors entered the field of electrical stimulation with the "Myofasciatron," the "Neuro-audio-palpator," and the "ever imitated" but "never duplicated" "Semi-Automatic White Light Instrument" built by Art Tool and Die of Detroit (fig. 8).[55]

Perhaps the most enduring electronic device originating from outside the profession was the Micro-Dynameter (fig. 9). Invented in the 1920s by F.C. Ellis, an engineering graduate from the University of Wisconsin, the impressive black and chrome instrument ostensibly diagnosed virtually every ailment by making the body function as a simple electrical cell and measuring the current generated. Variations from "normal" indicated problem areas. First, in a procedure "as simple as weighing," the operator determined the patient's "VITALITY," or electrochemical balance, by placing metal electrodes on the hands and feet to obtain a calibrated reading on the diagnostic scale. Next, the patient strapped a metal electrode to his or her forehead and was connected through the fingertips to the "polarimeter," an accessory device that measured patient "POLARITY." A normal individual exhibited neutral polarity, indicated by a "0" on the scale. Abnormal "displacements" to the right signified positive polarity; to the left, negative. From the combination of vitality and polarity, the Micro-Dynameter automatically calculated the precise dosage and type of current needed to restore the patient to a normal electrochemical balance. The operator then merely spun dials and clicked switches on the center panel.[56] To paraphrase Emerson, the operator sacrificed mother wit for machinery.[57]

Actually, the apparatus was a simple circuit known as a string galva-nometer and measured only the relative moisture of the patient's skin. It was marketed for more than three decades until the Food and Drug Administration (FDA) took Ellis Research Laboratories to federal court in 1962. During the trial, an FDA inspector explained that in a test the Micro-Dynameter had registered perfect health for two cadavers. The court found the device to be fraudulent and issued a condemnation order. When the FDA seized the machines, they found that more than 5,000 had been sold at prices ranging to $875.[58] Chiropractors were prominent among those duped by the Micro-Dynameter.

Harmonists and mechanics, straights and mixers, chiropractors and chiropractoids—the squabbles and schisms within chiropractic became legion. But disputes within medical sects, whether orthodox or unortho-dox, have been the historical rule. In the nineteenth century, regulars battled over the efficacy of heroic therapy while Thomsonians wrangled over the need for formal schooling in their art. Homeopaths split over the low dilution or high dilution of medicines while "lesion osteopaths" vied with "broad osteopaths" over the scope of practice.[59] Chiropractors were no different. Common interests do not automatically produce cooperation within groups. As medical sociologist Paul Starr has noted,

> it is easy to assume, as some analysts do, that because doctors, or any other group, share some imputed common interest . . . they will act coherently to support and defend that interest. Yet any number of factors—competing loyalties; internal conflicts; the inability of the members of a group or class to communicate with one another; the active hostility of the state, church, or other powerful institutions—can prevent the effective articulation of common interests.

At a minimum, according to Starr, collective action requires a way to induce members of a group to subordinate private affairs and contribute time and resources to the goals of the collective body. But common ends alone are insufficient inducement because organizational activities produce general benefits that, like common grace, fall on contributor and shirker alike. To counteract this "free ride" tendency and enlist participation, groups must provide "selective incentives"—benefits or penalties—other than the collective good.[60]

In the midst of their dissension, chiropractors slowly began to recognize that licensing laws were crucial for avoiding prosecution, crucial for the very survival and prosperity of their profession. State legislators were averse to granting licensing laws when chiropractors themselves failed to agree on a common definition of chiropractic. The need for licensing provided the selective incentives that pushed chiropractors toward collec-

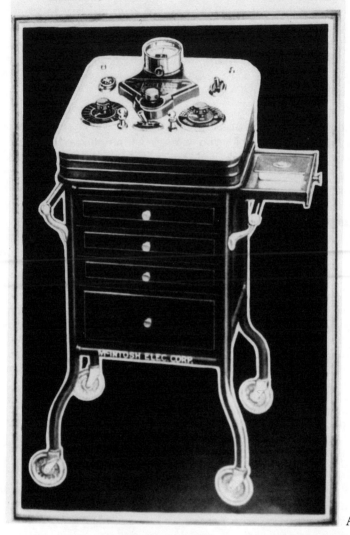

THE McINTOSH
"POLYSINE" GENERATOR
(Trade Mark Reg. U. S. Pat. Off.)   (Patent applied for)

A

FIGURE 7 (*A–D*). The Polysine Generator and its uses. From *Polysine Philosophy: The Story of the McIntosh Polysine Generator and Its Place in Physical Therapy Practice* (Chicago: McIntosh Electrical, 1929). A copy of this book is located in the Archives of the Logan College of Chiropractic, Chesterfield, Missouri.

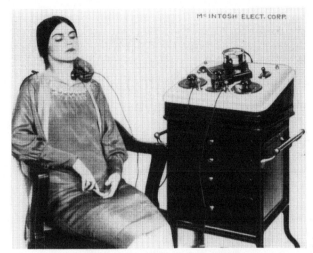

B

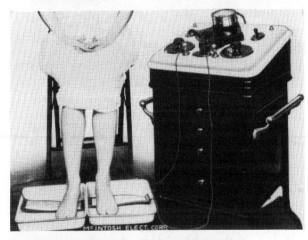

C

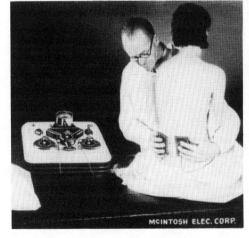

D

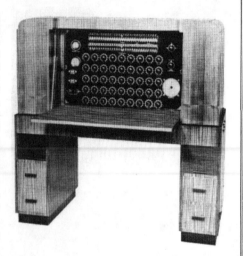
FIGURE 8. The Semi-Automatic White Light Instrument. From *The Chiropractic Journal*, c. 1930s. Courtesy of American Chiropractic Association.

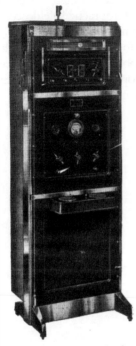
FIGURE 9. The Micro-Dynameter. From *The Chiropractic Journal,* c. 1930s. Courtesy of American Chiropractic Association.

tive action. Licensing held forth the promise and benefit of legitimacy; failing to reach the common ground needed for licensing meant the penalty of continued prosecution and the possibility of extinction.

Chiropractors bickered vigorously over what constituted true chiropractic, but all of the flecks and flickers in the chiropractic kaleidoscope, whether of a harmonial or a mechanical variety, turned within the circle of a drugless therapy, underwritten by Nature. In a drug-laden age, this common commitment provided the basis of cooperation for a fractured profession. The push for licensing helped chiropractors discover, as did Schopenhauer's porcupines, a mean distance of tolerable existence.

Chapter Four

The Chill of the Law

It has always been a sore in my eye to see how some who profess to be disciples of D.D. Palmer have tried and still insist on narrowing the science down to simple technic. In the early days it was necessary to protect the "child" (as D.D. was wont to refer to his Chiropractic) by evasive terminology in order to avoid the chill and ice of the law. . . . These terms were garments to protect the child until legal clothing could be secured.

Chiropractor John A. Howard, 1934

Medical society spokesman: "Yes, we are against you. We are against chiropractic and all other fakers. If this [New York] legislature will give us this bill, we will drive you and your ilk out of this state! What do you think about that?"

New York chiropractor Lyndon Lee: "First, sir, I'd like to see your driver's license."

Hearing in Albany, March 1926

Threatening skies halted the street march of their serenading brass band, so instead the score of well-wishers streamed into the warden's office of the Hudson County Jail in Jersey City on May 11, 1924, bearing chicken, baskets of fruit, candy, and flowers. They came in support of chiropractor J.H. Conover, who was serving the thirteenth day of a fifty-day sentence for practicing medicine without a license. "We are the patients of Dr. Conover," proclaimed a banner stretching across an automobile that brought them. "We want treatment." After a toast in his honor, Conover declared: "If the old-fashioned doctors want to put us out of business, let them make their patients well and that will force us to starve to death."[1]

Demonstrative grassroots sympathy for arrested chiropractors became commonplace across the country. Chiropractic patients frequently turned out for courtroom trials demanding acquittals and bearing witness of cures wrought by the hands of their indicted chiropractors. Convictions in jury trials were rare,[2] but if, as in Conover's case, the verdict meant jail, patients often paraded their support before the authorities. Chiropractors were quick to recognize the public relations value of spontaneous goodwill. At least two chiropractors in Texas, leaving little to chance, orchestrated processions celebrating their release from jail. In February 1922, Paul Meyers of Wichita Falls enlisted several patients to arrange his parade and himself posted bond and paid incidental expenses for the fifteen-block spectacle. After his self-directed parade, Byron L. Black of El Paso went on a chiropractic spree, adjusting all night long.[3]

"Practicing medicine without a license" became the ubiquitous charge leveled at chiropractors. With sixty-six cases filed against him, Charles C. Lemly of Waco, Texas, seems to hold the record. He suffered only one loss (his first trial), spent one hour in jail, and paid a ninety-five dollar fine. Joseph "Dr. Jodie" Baier was charged nineteen times his first year in Lufkin but continued an office practice with little interruption because the sympathetic sheriff would whistle for him out the courthouse window when his cases were called. Baier "would grab a spine and nerve chart and go to court. He was never convicted and usually got one or more members of the jury to come in for treatments later." James Riddle Drain, longtime president of Texas Chiropractic College, was even charged with "being about to practice medicine without a license," a case that was thrown out of court.[4]

To combat the allegations of practicing without a license, the defense typically called forth character recommendations from prominent citizens and solicited an impressive array of patient testimonials to reconstituted hearts, rejuvenated limbs, and reduced goiters. Michael S. Hogan, a Laurelton, Long Island, insurance agent, declared his intention in the *New York Journal and American* of February 16, 1939, to testify on behalf of indicted seventy-year-old chiropractor Frederick C. Zinke of Brooklyn "because he cured me of heart disease." According to Hogan, "sufferers are now being forced to 'bootleg' spinal adjustments to relieve heart, kidney, pulmonary, gastro-intestinal conditions, etc., but they do not let chiropractors down in case of arrest for practicing medicine without a license." The *Journal* correspondent closed the article by noting that "all of Chiropractor Zinke's patients will meet in the Brooklyn Academy of Music Sunday, to line up his defense."[5]

Casual readers of the article would probably assume that Zinke's backers represented an impromptu response to an imminent legal threat.

Actually, Zinke and Hogan had been involved for a decade with a highly organized group of laymen and practitioners devoted to fervent chiropractic boosterism. In 1927, Brooklyn chiropractor William H. Werner, a 1920 graduate of the Palmer School, had spearheaded the American Bureau of Chiropractic (ABC), formed, according to the platform, "to organize laymen to secure and maintain legal recognition of the science of chiropractic and its practitioners, to undertake a broad and intensive campaign to present chiropractic to the people, to gather and disseminate authentic information about the accomplishments of chiropractic, and to maintain a publicity bureau for the benefit of its members." One-hundred forty-five auxiliaries soon dotted the nation, with membership ranging from eight to several hundred members. Every chiropractor seemed to command his own lay bureau. In August 1930, the ABC held a joint convention in Davenport with the annual Palmer lyceum, energizing the affair by booming recorded testimony of chiropractic cures over the auditorium graphophone. A 1932 rally at Madison Square Garden drew over twelve thousand supporters. The movement soon spread to England, Canada, France, Belgium, Greece, and New Zealand—chiropractor Zinke rose to become the international treasurer and layman Hogan one of five international secretaries. "This zealous activity," wrote a contemporary sympathizer, "is an almost cult-like florescence such as might have sprung from the seeds of philosophy sown by D.D. Palmer. His teachings of the innate and educated intelligences, of vital energy—tone—and that both ancient and modern metaphysical argument woven about the theory, remain among this far-scattered but closely organized membership."[6]

Exuberant patient support was valuable but could carry the legally harassed chiropractor only so far. In addition, he needed an able defense. B.J. Palmer and his "straight" Universal Chiropractors Association retained the La Crosse, Wisconsin, firm of Morris & Hartwell as legal counsel after their successful defense in the Morikubo case of 1907. Thomas Morris's political prominence as a state senator and then lieutenant governor of Wisconsin helped to give the chiropractic cause a welcome measure of respectability. The chiropractic image was also aided when prominent local attorneys teamed with Morris. For example, in a 1918 trial in Dallas, Morris was assisted by Pat M. Neff, who later became governor of Texas and president of Baylor University.[7]

Morris and associates crisscrossed the country developing a canny defense while defending chiropractors in hundreds of cases. At Utica, Kansas, in 1911, Dr. Atwood, the local doctor of medicine, accused chiropractor Sadie Frank, a Palmer graduate, of practicing medicine without a license. Morris, heading the UCA defense for Frank, put Atwood on the stand.

Morris: Dr. Atwood, are you a licensed doctor?
Atwood: Yes, I am.
Morris: Do you take the Medical Journal and keep up on all the new treatments?
Atwood: Yes, I do.
Morris: Do you know what is meant by a specific remedy?
Atwood: Yes, according to my definition, I do know of such remedies.
Morris: Please state your definition.
Atwood: There are certain specific remedies for certain diseases, and for others we have no specific remedies. For these we try one thing and if that doesn't help, we try something else.

In his closing plea, Morris argued:

This man admits to you, the jury, that he doesn't know anything for sure. He will try some remedy for an illness, and if that doesn't restore health, he will try something else. Yet, he insists on you, the jury, to convict this lady of practicing medicine. Knowing those failures of medicine, she had the good judgment to choose a method which she studied in a school for that purpose, which method directs her attention to the nerve control of the organ in trouble. Is this not more scientific? Do you find it will be to your benefit, and the suffering public, to condemn this defendant because her method is not like that of medicine?

The jury returned a verdict of not guilty.[8] If, as Morris alleged, the therapeutic arsenal of orthodox, licensed physicians such as Atwood was simply the product of serendipity, penalizing the unorthodox and unlicensed held little justification.

"Go to Jail for Chiropractic"

Although the majority of arrested chiropractors were acquitted, many were convicted and willingly served jail terms as a testimony to their higher purpose of medical freedom. Hundreds of arrests in California in the decade before 1922 prompted the Federated Chiropractors of California to advise members to "Go to Jail for Chiropractic," a slogan that spread rapidly across the country and infused chiropractors with a sense of boldness and heroism. The Alameda County (California) Chiropractors' Association, organized in 1917, even required its members to choose a jail term rather than a fine if convicted.[9]

Instead of dampening the movement, the constant harassment of chiropractors by legal and medical authorities actually promoted chiropractic. Persecution bred sympathy and attendant publicity that increased business,[10] a common experience for the medical underdog in America. In the 1830s, for example, Thomsonians were beleaguered by courtroom maneuvers that proved largely fruitless. Samuel Thomson wrote in his

Narrative that the hounding of his botanical movement "has caused me a great deal of trouble and expense, and has been of no great benefit to them. It has been like whipping fire among the leaves, which only tends to spread it faster."[11] Later in the century, attempts by orthodox physicians to enforce the consultation clause of the American Medical Association code of ethics against homeopaths usually backfired. "If anything," historian Martin Kaufman explained, "persecution strengthened the will of the martyrs. It provided them with the moral assurance that they had something worth fighting to preserve. In addition, it brought them the sympathy of a public which cared little about medical theory."[12]

A jail term served further to radicalize the chiropractor, an experience that provided a second infilling of the chiropractic spirit as well as a badge of honor. There was no shame attached to the jail, and many chiropractors gave adjustments while imprisoned, converting both judges and jailers. "Going to Jail for Chiropractic" gave the chiropractor a personal witness, a moment of confrontation with the authorities, a personal, defiant act demonstrating his or her faith in the chiropractic idea (figs. 10 and 11). Texas chiropractor Marvin Bruce McCoy expressed a typical attitude when he defied the state's attorney general (who had vowed to chase chiropractors into the Gulf of Mexico) and was promptly arrested for practicing without a license: "Might surely was not on my side but I knew that Right was and I was ready to fight for it."[13] Still, the personal catharsis held potential danger for the movement if the need for witnessing became self-indulgent and more important than rectifying the perceived injustice lying behind the persecution.[14] However, the lure of legitimacy through licensing became stronger than the attraction of jail-cell martyrdom. A number of convictions in appellate courts alarmed many chiropractors into recognizing the need for licensing laws to establish chiropractic as a separate branch of the healing arts.[15] Going to jail had its limits. Even with licensing, continued charges of quackery would still offer enough persecution and martyrdom to go around.

Chiropractic existed in a legal nether world. Legislative redress through licensing became a necessary means of survival because chiropractors could not rely on courthouse maneuvers and judicial interpretations to exonerate them. Chiropractors clearly had violated the law if the practice of chiropractic was deemed to be the practice of medicine. The question of guilt hinged on this definition. From his jail cell in Scott County, Iowa, in 1906, D.D. Palmer himself had established the argument that chiropractors would follow for years to come. Chiropractic is not the practice of medicine, nor do chiropractors "desire to practice medicine, surgery or obstetrics," Palmer argued. Requiring healers who are not practicing medicine to undergo a four-year medical course to meet legal

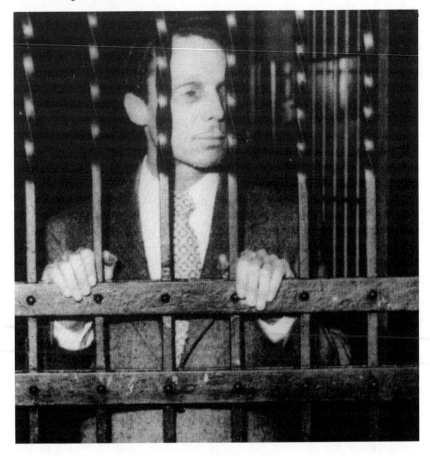

FIGURE 10. Chiropractor in prison: Herbert Reaver, sentenced to six months for practicing medicine without a license, 1947. Courtesy of *Chiropractic Achievers,* March/April 1989.

mandates is illogical. "Such requirements," he wrote in drawing a parallel between medical and religious freedom and implying the sectarian nature of regular medicine, "are no more just than it would be for the state to demand that all ministers should take a course of four years in a certain theological school before the applicant be allowed to preach the doctrines of another sect whose views were dramatically opposite." Such an imposition, he held, would surely "warp" the student's original intent.[16]

Was chiropractic the practice of medicine? Subsequent laws and court rulings were frequently contradictory. Individual state statutes prohibiting

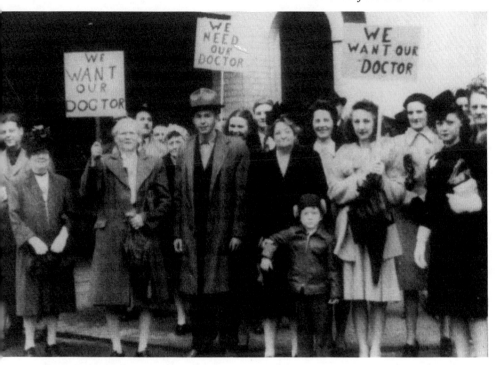

FIGURE 11. Patients demonstrate for the release of Herbert Reaver, 1947.
Courtesy of *Chiropractic Achievers,* March/April 1989.

the unlicensed practice of medicine largely determined whether chiropractic
fell under the rubric of "medicine." Where a statute defined medical practice
in broad terms, the courts have interpreted chiropractic as violating the
law. In 1915, the Supreme Judicial Court of Massachusetts found Boston
chiropractor J.O. Zimmerman guilty of violating chapter 76, section 8 of
the 1902 Revised Laws of the state, which penalized the unauthorized
practitioner with a fine or a fine and imprisonment. In Commonwealth v.
Zimmerman,[17] Chief Justice Rugg argued that medicine encompasses a
"broad field," relating to "the prevention, cure and alleviation of disease,
the repair of injury, or treatment of abnormal or unusual states of the body
and their restoration to a healthful condition" and is "not confined to
the administering of medicinal substances or the use of surgical or other
instruments." Even if a practitioner devotes himself only to a "very restricted" part of the field, "he still may be found to practice medicine."
That Zimmerman described his methods as analysis, palpation, and adjustment and refrained from using the terms *diagnosis, treatment,* or *disease*

failed to impress the court. Substance rather than style was the issue; chiropractic was the practice of medicine.

The court was also unimpressed with a harmonial wrinkle developed only after the adverse decision of the lower, Suffolk County court. Zimmerman's attorneys argued before the Supreme Judicial Court that the defendant fell within the exceptions to section 8 detailed in section 9 of the Revised Laws, expressly the last provision exempting from penalty those who practiced the "cosmopathic method of healing." Chief Justice Rugg turned to his dictionary to define *cosmopathic* as "open to the access of supernormal knowledge or emotion supposedly from a preternatural world." In a display of legal obliquity, Rugg then refused to undertake a definition of what a cosmopathic method might entail but still contended that "plainly, it does not include the defendant's operations." Whether Zimmerman qualified as cosmopathic or not was actually a moot point at law. As Rugg explained, because Zimmerman had failed in the lower court to claim any exceptions within section 9, the point could no longer be saved.[18]

Zimmerman also challenged the constitutionality of the statute by claiming that chiropractic was denied equal protection of the law through unreasonable classification because section 9 exempted certain classes of healers (such as osteopaths, pharmacists, mind curists, masseurs, and Christian Scientists) from the medical examination required by section 8. The court dismissed this contention by noting that the constitutionality of the statute in question was already affirmed by previous decisions[19] and that the "rational classification" of healers rightly fell within the power of the legislature and could not be overthrown by the facts of the present case. Because chiropractic was defined as the practice of medicine, the Zimmerman decision meant, curiously, that only licensed doctors of medicine could practice chiropractic legally. Commonwealth v. Zimmerman established an important precedent, often cited in future cases, and seriously hampered the development of chiropractic in Massachusetts. Not until 1966, when Governor Volpe reluctantly signed a chiropractic licensing bill, did the profession successfully hurdle a half-century of legal obstacles in the state.[20]

In sharp contrast to the Zimmerman decision, at least ten state supreme courts held that drugless healing was not the practice of medicine. Typically, the statutes of these states defined medical practice in narrower terms than in Massachusetts, as limited to one who prescribed any drug, medicine, or other agency.[21] The ambiguity of "other agency" was usually resolved by applying the rule of *ejusdem generis*,[22] interpreted in a restrictive sense to mean another agency similar to drug or medicine. A number of rulings in these states were decidedly sympathetic to chiropractic. In Norman v. Hastings (1920), Judge Lansden wrote for the Supreme Court of Tennessee that "the Court thinks that Chiropractors cannot be classed along with Charlatans and fakirs. This science of healing is well developed and recognized in many jurisdictions and many believe in its efficacy. It is not suggested on the record that the practice of the science is in any way deleterious to the human body."[23] In People v. Love (1921), Justice W.W. Duncan delivered the opinion of the Illinois Supreme Court, noting that "the prejudice existing against chiropractors by medical men and osteopaths is known to be intense and in many cases very unreasonable." The Love decision reversed the judgment of the Vermilion County Court by holding that section 22 of the Medical Practice Act of 1917 violated both section 1, article 2 of the Constitution of Illinois and the due process clause of the fourteenth amendment of the federal Constitution. The Medical Practice Act prescribed that an applicant for the unlimited practice of medicine and surgery be a graduate of a "reputable" medical college without specifying a particular length of study but required an applicant for a license to practice drugless healing without operative surgery to complete a four-year course of instruction in an institution offering the system he desired to practice. The court held the statute unconstitutional because it "unlawfully and unjustly" discriminated against one class of physicians for no discernible reason by requiring that the professional education of limited practitioners be of greater duration than that for those with an unlimited scope of practice. In addition, the court ruled that a regulation of the Department of Registration and Education obligating chiropractors to submit letters of recommendation from at least two reputable medical men or osteopaths along with their application for examination was "arbitrary and unreasonable" and that submission to such a mandate would in all probability result in exclusion from examination.[24] Although the Love decision stood as a resounding victory for chiropractors it was, like their practice, limited in scope. The court was careful to note that it could only determine discriminatory features of existing acts; the proper length of professional education and the qualifications of practitioners were solely legislative matters. Chiropractors could not depend on judicial interpretations to stamp the vocation with legitimacy. An appeal to state legislatures for regulation through chiropractic licensing laws seemed to be the only safe route to survival.

MEDICAL REGULATION IN AMERICA

When it became clear to chiropractors that they could not escape the strictures of the law through judicial interpretation, they agitated for "friendly" licensing laws that would give them autonomous examining boards. Only licensing that allowed chiropractors to direct their own affairs would ensure survival. The push for chiropractic licensing became part of a broader wave of occupational licensing initiated in the late nineteenth century, which finally institutionalized medical regulation in America after more than two centuries of sporadic and largely ineffective efforts. For chiropractors, as for all medical purveyors in the twentieth century, licensing became a crucial step toward legitimacy.

At common law, anyone with medical pretensions could minister to the sick, liable only for damages in cases of malpractice and subject to the right of government to exclude incompetents by *quo warranto*.[25] In a vague statute in 1649, the Massachusetts General Court first attempted to regulate the ministrations of "Chirurgeons, Midwives, Physitians or others," those "imployed . . . about the bodye of men, women or children, for preservation of life, or health." A provision requiring the aspiring practitioner to secure the advice and consent of the medically skillful proved ineffective. The practice of physic remained open to all; more than a century would elapse before additional regulatory efforts were undertaken at the provincial level.[26]

In America, British guild distinctions among physicians (university graduates addressed as "doctor"), surgeons (considered craftsmen and addressed as "mister"), and apothecaries (compounders and sellers of drugs) were easily ignored in the absence of licensing regulations, especially where a scattered, frontier population encouraged domestic practice and provided only part-time work for the would-be doctor.[27] In the colonies, it was easy to move from cobbling boots to cobbling bodies. Empirics frequently entered the field, often after news of a remarkable cure traveled the circuits of local gossip. Some American doctors in the eighteenth century learned their medical skills through the apprentice system and were admitted to practice solely at the pleasure of their preceptors. Such "training," however, had little, if any, connection to effective healing. Citizens frequently noted the woeful state of medical care and agitated for regulation that would bring some order to medical practice. Although historian William Smith's oft-quoted lamentation (*History of the Province of New York*, 1757) applies an Old World standard to the colonies and confuses training with skill and empiricism with quackery, it nevertheless describes an important, contemporary perception: "Few physicians among us are eminent for their skill. Quacks abound like locusts in Egypt. This is less to be wondered at as the profession is under no kind of Regulation. Any man at his pleasure sets up for Physician, Apothecary, and Chirurgen."[28]

In 1760, the Provincial Assembly of New York passed the first colonial act requiring examination for licensing. The statute provided both a nonmedical board of examiners and penalties for unlicensed practice but applied only to New York City and enforcement was lax. In 1772, the provincial legislature of New Jersey enacted a similar, colony-wide law, with authority vested in the New Jersey Medical Society. Between 1780 and 1830, most states followed the New Jersey precedent by establishing some type of licensing procedure with state and local medical societies operating as licensing agencies. The societies soon clashed with administrators of medical schools, who assumed that a degree automatically conferred the right to practice. The convention of requiring either a medical degree or examination before the board as a condition for licensing developed in most areas after the Massachusetts Medical Society agreed in 1803 to accept a Harvard medical degree in place of examination. Yet the system rarely deterred unlicensed practitioners. The basic distinction between the licensed and the unlicensed was the right of the licensed to sue for uncollected fees, an honorific right that often meant little in practice. The threat of fines on the unlicensed proved hollow, since imposition required the verdict of a (frequently reluctant) jury. After 1830, however, state after state repealed even these ineffective penalties on unlicensed healers, primarily because the concept of licensure offended a growing democratic impulse suspicious of elite control and special privilege. At a time when regular, licensed physicians lacked therapies superior to those of irregulars, their cries that licensing upheld science against quackery were unconvincing. Unorthodox practitioners, led by the Thomsonian botanics, argued for free competition that relied on the common sense of a competent public against medical monopoly, a cry that chiropractors would often advance a hundred years later in arguing *for* chiropractic licensing in an era when licensure had reemerged and was firmly entrenched. For chiropractors, free competition would mean licensing any group that could demonstrate therapeutic effectiveness and command devotion among the public. But in a Jacksonian world, medical licenses seemed to confer favor rather than signal competence; medical societies loomed merely as closed corporations similar to banks and other monopolies. In addition, licenses meant little when a burgeoning number of proprietary schools churned out graduates by the hundreds who practiced by virtue of holding a degree. By the time of the Civil War, no state retained an effective licensing law.[29]

Uncontrolled entry into medicine continued until states and territories began to reenact licensure laws in the 1870s, spurred by stronger state medical societies crying out for improvement in medical education. In his American Medical Association (AMA) presidential address in 1883, Dr. N.S. Davis did not argue for returning licensing power to state societies but urged the societies to lobby their legislators for state control that would wrest power away from medical schools.[30] Inferior and bogus schools would abound as long as a degree alone conferred the right of practice. Ironically, the first wave of medical practice acts in most states required only that a registrant present a medical college diploma, a demand that promoted medical diploma mills rather than forcing them from business. Of forty-one states and territories that began licensing before 1890, thirty-four issued licenses to degree holders without further proof of fitness. Gradually, states amended their laws by requiring all applicants to pass board examinations and discriminated between schools by imposing escalating standards for curriculum length and content on the applicants' medical colleges. By 1910, every state had a medical board with power to judge the quality of medical degrees and all mandated at least a three-year curriculum. Therefore, the famous Flexner Report of 1910 had little immediate effect on licensure laws except to spur laggard states to catch up.[31]

The push to license physicians was actually part of a larger movement of occupational licensing in the late nineteenth century, a new wave intent on professionalization that exalted expert, specialized knowledge. Recent historians have grappled with the problems of defining the term *profession* and the reasons behind this late nineteenth century passion for professionalism. In *The Professions in American History,* Nathan O. Hatch observed that definitions of what constitutes a profession "multiply without end" but usually involve three classic criteria: a definable body of organized knowledge accompanied by expertise derived from specialized academic training; a moral commitment to public service that extends beyond a desire for personal gain (the professional "does not work in order to be paid but is paid in order to work"); and a relative autonomy within professional life.[32]

But this definition seems a little too tidy. In addition to practitioners with their specialized education, Bruce Sinclair noted that a profession also involves decidedly social and political, intramural aspects—organizations, meetings, transactions, definitions of intellectual style, and codes of conduct. Michael Schudson added the criterion that "honorable" and "respected" professions (read "true" professions?) are those that treat ultimate concerns, such as life and death (doctors), liberty and justice (lawyers), and transcendent matters (clergyman), returning full circle to the three, age-old, venerable professions.[33]

In the midst of this sociological and historical confusion, Laurence Veysey threw up his hands and asked that the effort to arrive at an abstract definition of the term *professional* be abandoned. Professions, he argued, should be defined "as nothing more than a series of rather random occupations that have historically been called that in our own culture (recognizing that the occupations thought appropriate to the label have changed over time), and that have conferred at least fairly high social status on their practitioners and their families, while demanding some kind of extended training, usually—though not always—in universities." Still, Veysey continued, it should be remembered that poets do not seem to require the "professional" label, even though they possess word skills at least equal with those of lawyers.[34]

Despite the difficulty of arriving at a comprehensive definition of profession, turn-of-the-century Americans seemed obsessed with professionalism and its accoutrements. In *The Culture of Professionalism,* Burton Bledstein argued that a "conceptual revolution" among middle class Americans created a distinctive culture of ceremonies and rituals (enshrined in the newly emerging university) which cultivated elitist tendencies often found in democracies. According to Bledstein, Americans invented universities to sanction success based presumably on merit and objectivity rather than class or heredity, a system that minted a new elite still consonant with democratic ideology. Professionalization provided a framework for creating orderly, authoritative explanations within a society that tended to reject traditional authority. The structuring of space coupled with the use of special words (e.g., in classrooms, courtrooms, and hospitals) was a crucial part of this professionalization and pushed devotees of a broad range of activities, from bicycling to barbering, to elevate their particular interests to the status of profession.[35] A late nineteenth-century world where housekeeping becomes home economics and where public health officials rhapsodize over the scientific status of the plumber[36] is only a short, conceptual step away from a late twentieth-century world where elevator operators are members of the "vertical transportation corps," car mechanics are "automotive internists," gas station attendants are "petroleum transfer engineers," paper boys are "media couriers," department store guards are "Loss Prevention Specialists," and potato chip delivery truck drivers are "Executive Snack Route Consultants."[37] Professionalism, as Robert Dingwall noted, is the peculiar "Anglo-Saxon disease."[38]

According to Thomas Haskell in *The Emergence of Professional Social Science,* the key to understanding this inclination toward professionalism is the growing awareness among nineteenth-century Americans of a highly interdependent social universe. The history of the American Social Science Association provided him with a vehicle for understanding three general problems associated with this emerging modern consciousness: the "crisis" of professional authority; the "growing persuasiveness" of the turn-of-the-century professional social-science practitioners; and the "decisive reorientation of social thought" that occurred in the 1890s. Haskell argued that the context of professionalization (that he believed other scholars have misunderstood) was the movement to solidify authority in both the intellectual and moral realms. Postbellum adherents of the Social Science Association moved in a world of independent action, a world where the individual was still potent and where cause and effect, explanation and prediction seemed to be relatively simple matters. In the rapidly industrializing and urbanizing world of the late century, however, growing interdependence created a world of flux. "Where all is *inter*dependent," Haskell explained, "there can be no '*in*dependent' variables." Only painstaking and exhaustive research can begin to reveal cause and effect in even a tentative way. This complex, difficult task by necessity falls to specialists, a business outside the realm of public opinion. The creation of professional institutions, then, became a way to give each audience within the public its own worthy and authoritative guide.[39]

Chiropractic, emerging at the end of the century during this time of cultural transformation, offended this growing sensibility of interdependence by clinging to older patterns of causation. For the first generation of chiropractors, the cause of disease (subluxated vertebrae) was clear, and adjustment would create the desired effect (health). If professionalization meant presiding over an increasingly complex and interdependent world, then early chiropractors had no use for the concept. The Palmers and their harmonial followers wanted to be recognized for possessing Truth, not simply for having an expert skill. The argument within chiropractic was over whether or not chiropractic was indeed a profession or even should be. B.J. Palmer and his harmonial followers sought to keep his father's invention in the older empiricist tradition, a tradition that depended on inspiration and messianic genius. Mechanics within chiropractic wanted to professionalize along the newer models of systematic knowledge and conform to definitions developing within medicine. For the Palmers to follow this path would mean giving up claims to special genius and allowing, in effect, a democratization of chiropractic. Ironically, professionalization for chiropractic would serve to *broaden* the movement rather than constrict it because becoming an expert was easy. The courts (a forum in which public opinion as expressed through jurors still counted heavily) also served to promote this democratization because they had such difficulty distinguishing clearly among medical experts and their claims. The parodies of modern scientific technology employed after minimal training by second-generation chiropractors, along with degrees such as the D.C. (Doctor of Chiropractic) and the Ph.C. (Philosopher of Chiropractic), helped chiropractors project a "professional" image that blurred distinctions between chiropractors and other medical experts who also used new-fashioned technology to treat the ill. Everyman (even through the mail) could become a chiropractor, outfitted with the trappings of the medical professional. Chiropractic, then, provides a counterexample to historians, such as Bledstein and Haskell, who have emphasized the exclusionary social implications of professionalization.

By the time chiropractors were emerging in ever-increasing numbers during the second decade of the century, licensure was rooted firmly. The new laws, however, did not mean that orthodox physicians had become a powerful interest group. Regulars had sought cooperation from homeopaths and eclectics in order to obtain legislation. A new pattern of "friendly" licensing evolved; regulations were sought and enforced by practitioners themselves and required only moderate licensing fees. The older pattern had been intentionally hostile, enforced by local officials demanding high fees (e.g., for peddler licenses) and designed to restrict competition with established tradesmen. In a changed economic landscape where large corporations increasingly dominated, friendly licensing became a way for the independent, struggling businessman to survive and to strike back. Licensing in the Jacksonian era had been identified with privilege, but by the turn of the century it became a weapon for the small-time operator to wield against regnant corporations and a means of survival for the threatened.[40] Before, freedom meant repealing licensure; now it meant acquiring it.

Tightening controls in the medical practice acts began to transform them from friendly to increasingly hostile in intent. Yet chiropractors needed friendly licensing laws that granted them autonomy in developing their discipline, freedom that regulators were reticent to permit. In arguing their case for autonomy, chiropractors claimed, in effect, that the medical profession was acting as a dominant corporation that sought unjustly to snuff out competition by denying them licensing altogether or, as a last resort, by enforcing hostile licensing that would place chiropractors under the control of a board dominated by medical doctors. Chiropractors knew that just any licensing law wouldn't do; the wrong type would spell disaster. The power to license was also the power to destroy.

MEDICAL FREEDOM AND THE PUBLIC INTEREST: CHIROPRACTIC LICENSING IN AMERICA

In *The Governmental Process*, the classic study of interest group politics, David Truman noted that, "where there is any real possibility of materially extending the dimensions of a given public, the group that expects to benefit must usually be able to identify itself with some widely held objective even though the immediate benefits of the advocated legislation will be narrowly distributed."[41] For chiropractors, proper licensing would serve the larger ideals of medical freedom and, even more broadly, uphold freedom and the right of choice itself. Philip Troupe, a staunch chiropractic advocate and editor of the *New Haven* (Conn.) *Union News*, roused his audience at the Chiropractors' Convention of the East in Atlantic City on June 22, 1924, by reminding them that their current legislative battles were part of the age-old "nobility of higher purposes," selfless acts transcending the immediate issues:

> It is not a very far cry . . . , between the spirit of a man who says to another—
> "You believe as I do about God and what is good for your soul or I shall persecute you!" and the one who says—"You believe as I do about what is good for your body or I will imprison you!" [applause]

So my friends, we are on the threshold of another great battle for human liberty and you people who represent Chiropractic should get on the firing line. There are two sides lined up as always. . . .
Chiropractic is bigger than any individual in it; bigger than any school that represents it; bigger than all the schools that represent it. [applause] It is the truth and nothing is bigger than truth![42]

In opposing the spread of chiropractic, osteopathy, Christian Science, and the other healing groups, the regular profession identified *its* motive as safeguarding the public interest. Perhaps the most colorful expression of this ideal came in 1906 when the New York state legislature was considering passage of an osteopathic law. Abraham Jacobi, a German immigrant and future AMA president, brought laughter from the crowded gallery when he proclaimed in a thick accent, "Vat ve vant is to veed them all oudt so they cannot humbug the public for ve know how easy it is to humbug the public."[43] Two decades later, the public interest was still in peril according to Dr. Louis I. Harris, Commissioner of Public Health for New York City. "The ever-increasing threat of cults and quacks is like a hydra-headed monster," Harris warned. "You destroy one and others rise up against you. It is a preposterous spectacle to see the medical profession always on the aggressive to prevent a host of these persons from jimmying their way into the realm of medicine."[44]

Actually, both orthodox and unorthodox practitioners have acted frequently as trade associations, operating under the banner of the "public interest." However fervently the ideals may be held, the concept of an inclusive "public interest" fails to describe any real situation within a complex nation. As David Truman has argued, claims of serving a national or public interest become a convenient and often effective rhetorical device for a particularly extensive group to weaken or eliminate opposing interests. But a single public interest is nonexistent; groups compete in a world composed of many publics. To countermand the assertions of a pervasive group, an opposing body must expand its public by elevating its purpose from self-interest to altruism. Propaganda, always referred to as "educational" or "informational" work by the sponsoring group, provides a major way of communicating purposes and mobilizing support among potential allies. Chiropractor Lyndon Lee argued for a concerted, professional public relations initiative to advance the cause: "Public Information! Propaganda, if you will, but not the distorted thing we have come to know as propaganda. We should employ that form of propaganda which is the dissemination of truth. Dignified, of course; truthful, most certainly; but vigorous, continuous and widespread." Chiropractic should exploit the methods of modern advertising, Lee noted. "Our science must become as familiar to the public as that product which is 'Good to the last drop,' or the one which invites us to 'Ask the man who owns one,' or those which are known to us as the '57 Varieties.' Hardly a person will fail to recognize each of these."[45]

The propagandist has the greatest advantage with the audience when offering explanations for ambiguous events. People need clarification when the meaning of an event is unclear and are receptive to a sensible interpretation. "Such conditions often provide opportunities for groups otherwise at a disadvantage," Truman explained, "since established standards of judgment no longer adequately account for experience."[46] Chiropractic propaganda has had just such an advantage because back pain is usually a baffling event that the regular profession is frequently unable to explain or treat effectively. For many, chiropractors clarified the reason for pain and in the process identified their vocation as serving the ideals of freedom and liberty, ideals that few fail to laud.

Chiropractors could readily agree on the seat of pain as well as the larger purposes of their calling, but not on the precise language of licensing laws that would ensure the ideals of medical freedom. B.J. Palmer and his harmonial followers were not completely convinced that licensing insured their freedom because licensing laws required that chiropractic be defined; limitation is the nature of definition and clear definition would have the effect of constricting B.J.'s leadership. Any limitation tended to hamper development of the "high" science of a dynamic chiropractic, especially the "S. P. & U." (specific, pure, and unadulterated) or "straight" variety that B.J. was constantly evolving through the introduction of novel modalities and fresh techniques. In contrast, the mechanics and assorted "mixers" within chiropractic were willing to assume the role of back specialist and incorporate this reduced status within the language of the law. B.J. knew that the greatest battle for legislation would be the intramural skirmish over definition and warned his brethren to guard against so-called chiropractors who would sell the vocation at discount. The medical doctor is not the greatest enemy, he told the New York State Chiropractic Society in November 1915.

> Let it be understood, when it comes to getting legislation; he is not our worst enemy by any means. The worst enemy is the chiropractor. . . . Let it be understood squarely as you go into this work you will find your worst fight will come from chiropractors, so-called, who will not unite with you. And that if it centers to this ultimate end and the legislature finds you are split, you as the man who is a chiropractor and the other one who calls himself such—of course you must remember the legislature does not know the difference—he says you are split, you don't know what you want, when you don't know what you want how can you expect us to know what to give you.[47]

Despite such bickering, chiropractors were able to join loosely in pushing legislation through most of the states. In 1913, Kansas became the first to enact a chiropractic statute (although North Dakota was the first actually to issue a chiropractic license)[48] and, before 1920, thirteen additional states followed. In the decade of the twenties alone, twenty-five states and the District of Columbia passed chiropractic licensing laws, and by 1938 all but seven states had some type of legislative provision for chiropractic (see appendix A). Perhaps the most amusing political maneuver came in the midthirties in Texas after chiropractors complained that the medically slanted public health committee never gave chiropractic bills any real consideration. One unfriendly legislator suggested, "Why don't we refer it to the Livestock Committee with the rest of the jackasses?" When chiropractic lobbyists replied that the livestock committee would be preferable to the public health committee, the bill went to livestock. It was voted out of committee for consideration by the whole legislature, but got no further.[49]

The 1920s witnessed the greatest number of chiropractic laws by far. In the postwar era, the Progressive reformers' earlier assumption of an omnicompetent sovereign citizen, rational and capable, was crumbling. Widespread use of intelligence testing during the war indicated that the average citizen was deficient in basic intelligence and might be incapable of rational choice. (Harvard psychologist Robert M. Yerkes administered his Army Mental Tests to 1.75 million recruits during World War I and determined the average mental age of white American adults to be 13.08 years, barely a year above the level of "moron").[50] The laws and regulations of the Progressive era, such as the 1906 Pure Food and Drugs Act, were based on the assumption that the average person could direct his or her own course if the risks were made apparent. In the 1920s, such an assumption seemed incredibly naive. Laws and regulations would need to do more than simply provide reliable information; they would need to constrict the range of choice so that the selections of a credulous public would be safe. In this atmosphere, the enactment of chiropractic licensing laws became the only way to serve both the ideals of medical freedom and the public interest. Whether the licensing laws were friendly or hostile to chiropractic, the intention was to protect a public susceptible to propaganda and no longer able to act competently in its own behalf.

What chiropractors wanted, in effect, were friendly licensing laws that allowed them an autonomous chiropractic licensing board with total independence from state medical and educational authorities. For chiropractors, osteopathic legislation became a principle object lesson in what to avoid. Osteopaths had frequently allowed composite boards and had permitted educational control from outside the profession. Chiropractors saw this, with considerable justification, as a successful ploy by medical doctors to absorb and ultimately destroy chiropractic, as they had osteopathy. The January 1921 *New York State Journal of Medicine* proclaimed: "If we amend the Medical Practice Act so that no matter what a man wants to practice, whether it be Chiropractic or any other thing, he can do so provided he passes the same examination in other things as we do, it will be a good thing for the profession. You know we eliminated the osteopath when we made the General Medical Examining Board and put an Osteopath on it." In a message of caution to the 1925 graduating class of the Standard School of Chiropractic, Lyndon Lee warned that, since 1907, when osteopathy in New York came under medical control, only two osteopathic institutions had received recognition under the medical law and that these two institutions had produced fewer than seventy-five licensed graduates in the previous seventeen years.[51]

"Compromise legislation" became the bête noire of chiropractic and displayed several features, singly or in combination: composite boards with chiropractors in the minority, basic science laws requiring applicants first to pass science examinations, a board of regents setting educational standards or another extrachiropractic body establishing both the entrance requirements and the length of chiropractic courses, and statutes that revoked licenses if the chiropractor advertised.[52]

Yet chiropractors were not always able to enact ideal legislation, and in some states they settled for certain "compromise," hostile features as the price of legalization. Arkansas, Connecticut, Minnesota, Nebraska, Washington, Wisconsin, and the District of Columbia were the first to require chiropractic applicants to pass basic science tests in subjects such as physiology, pathology, and chemistry and in some cases in bacteriology, toxicology, and diagnosis, with answers judged from the orthodox viewpoint.[53] By 1946, eighteen states had established basic science boards to conduct examinations, scrutiny that had the effect of excluding chiropractors from these states. Between 1929 and 1950, for example, no chiropractor was able to pass Nebraska's Basic Science Board and by 1965 there were only seventy licensed chiropractors in the state. A 1957 change in the Kansas law requiring the science test for licensure had the clear consequence of closing the state to new chiropractors.[54]

Measured against medical and osteopathic examinees, chiropractors fared poorly on basic science boards. From 1927 to 1944, 87 percent of some twenty thousand medical students passed the exams, whereas only 28 percent of the 367 chiropractors succeeded.[55] From 1945 to 1953, 85 percent of 27,242 medical doctors and 67.4 percent of 2,461 osteopaths who sat for the boards passed, compared with only 21.9 percent of 2,202 chiropractic examinees.[56] Cash Asher, onetime public relations director of both the National and the International Chiropractic Associations, denounced basic science laws as the "death potion" for chiropractic. "With the awkward grace of a baboon putting on a tuxedo," Asher complained, "chiropractors are slipping into the straight-jacket of basic science laws.

The jacket does not fit any better than the tux fits the baboon, but Dr. Average Chiropractor shoves his hands and arms into the sleeve while trying to hold his nose against the odor of drugs about the garment."[57]

Indiana, New Jersey, and West Virginia also proved to be difficult states for chiropractic applicants because of composite boards with physician members outnumbering chiropractors. Colorado, Illinois, and Virginia provided no distinct chiropractic board and granted chiropractic licenses only through state medical boards without chiropractic representation.[58] For decades, legislators in New York, Massachusetts, Mississippi, and Louisiana resisted the tide of chiropractic licensing, but by 1974 all fifty states had passed chiropractic licensure laws.[59]

In July 1963, after the "Great Backward State of New York" had at last capitulated and enacted licensure following a protracted and embittered fifty-year battle, Lyndon Lee wrote to a patient who had congratulated him on the long-sought legislation.

> To be sure we, chiropractors, have been the active agents carrying forward the legislative work, but really it is you and thousands of other loyal patients who have made the success possible. At long last it was impressed on the Governor and the authorities in Albany that people were patronizing chiropractors in increasing numbers, and were growing more resentful at the refusal to establish the work on a properly controlled basis. This public sentiment finally had its effect.[60]

Although patient support was vital, Lee had understated the role of the practitioners themselves. Chiropractic fervor and tenacity in the face of perennial disappointment and harassment became a hallmark of chiropractors across the nation, a legacy of temperament descending from the Palmers. To endure the chill of the law and the charge of quackery required a certain disposition, an attitude of mission that elevated personal struggle to the level of righteous cause. The chiropractic ranks were filled with missionaries who willed the survival of their chosen calling.

Chapter Five

Missionaries of Health

*Is it not, then, actually a part of our duty—as missionaries of health—
to acquaint the people with the health-giving possibilities open to them
through chiropractic?*

Lyndon Lee

*We sing a song of rev'rence, of love and loyalty
To Chiropractic pioneers, We sing to honor Thee.
So here's to men of vision, We dedicate our all,
The Chiropractic brotherhood will answer to your call.*

*We pour out our devotion, May service be our aim
We give of all our courage, We work to bring-u-fame
Of Chiropractic wonders we'll never cease to sing
May each and ev'ry countryside with Chiropractic ring.*

D.L. Dennis, "An Ode to the Chiropractor"

*If anything ail a man so that he does not perform his functions, if he
have a pain in his bowels even . . . he forthwith sets about reforming—
the world.*

Henry David Thoreau

CONVERTING TO CHIROPRACTIC

In late 1910, chiropractor Mary Deneen told a gathering at the Palmer School of her work in the school clinic, how day after day she watched tears of pain turn to tears of joy as chiropractic relieved sickness and suffering. One lady, Deneen reported, told her how she hated to leave: "It's been a heaven to me, full of health and happiness, and you make me feel like this is one large family, full of filial love. I have not felt so good for fifteen years, as I have my short stay here." Most who came, Deneen continued, held little hope of relief because "their sentence had already been passed upon by the M.D.'s" who had them preparing for death. "How could you expect them to believe it when our faculty would tell them they could soon throw their crutches away and go rejoicing?" Yet after daily adjustments for a few short weeks, skepticism melted into gratitude and they went out "to proclaim the glad news of Chiropractic, as did the first."[1]

Such deliverance from a pain-wracked life, dramatic and compelling, often prompted a profound conversion to a way of health that not only sent converts into the streets proclaiming the glad news, but also convinced many to abandon their current livelihood and take up a chiropractic career as a means of testifying and ministering more directly to their newfound Way of Health.[2] These "work-weary plumbers and retired piano movers," as H.L. Mencken lampooned them, were perhaps easy to make sport of, but most *had* experienced relief from chiropractic after medical failure had left them in despair. In April 1942, Ronald McCurdy, age eight, tossed a two-inch-long strip of metal into the air as he lay listening to the radio and inadvertently swallowed it when it fell into his mouth. The piece proved to be too large for physicians to bring back up through the throat, and surgical removal was thwarted when the metal lodged itself in the cecum, the sac that begins the large intestine. Next-door neighbor and chiropractor A.L. Nickson then began daily treatments and with "Basic Technique" was able to move the metal into the large intestine, where nature accomplished the elimination forty-five days after the swallowing (fig. 12).[3]

That chiropractic frequently became a final, last-ditch hope after a string of medical disappointments actually benefited the movement in important ways. Because most cases chiropractors handled had not re-sponded to an orthodox approach, a type of automatic winnowing took effect that unwittingly became a prescription for chiropractic success. A patient with an organic problem (largely outside the realm of chiropractic effectiveness) would probably experience some relief from the chemical or surgical approach of his medical doctor and never seek out a chiropractor. But a mechanical problem that manipulation *could* ease would likely baffle the physician and send the frustrated patient searching for alternatives. Because chiropractors saw patients whose ailments were largely predis-posed to a chiropractic solution, their lack of training and proficiency in diagnosing disease became little hindrance to success. When chiropractors did help their patients, the relief appeared all the more remarkable because previous, orthodox procedures had failed. Such miraculous cures bred an understandable zealousness for the wonders of chiropractic. For example, in a "Testimonial Questionnaire" dated February 17, 1955, patient Florence M. Lindner of Creve Coeur, Missouri, testified to her new-found faith.

Once upon a time I had been one of those smug individuals who felt the M.D.s were infallible and that the chiropractors were really a group of quacks who "popped" bones and preyed upon the ignorant.

Truly I was the ignorant [one] for I did not understand the science of chiropractic.

And then came colitis and many costly visits to the M.D.s and to the hospital. I consumed drug upon drug including opium which they prescribed along with the other sedatives. All to no avail. My entire nervous system was effected [*sic*] by these many drugs. In fact, but for divine providence I might have become a dope addict quite innocently thru medical prescription. When I terminated my treatment from the medical profession and started my chiropractic treatment and stopped the drug consumption, only then I realized how horribly my nervous system was being affected by drugs.

When I visited my M.D. the last time he told me I would always be the victim of colitis—that one doesn't ever lick colitis.

But my chiropractor proved otherwise. I have one sincere hope that chiropractic will be preserved and that the medical profession will some day cooperate and know its benefits.[4]

The impact of chiropractic failure, on the other hand, was blunted if the patient reasoned that, after all, regular doctors had also disappointed. Only if chiropractors actively harmed their patients were they open for censure and subject to abuse. Sometimes such failure could erupt into violent acts by disgruntled patients. In May 1924, New Jersey chiropractor George A. Nelson died with a fractured skull after John Vollmer, a patient in his home, dealt him seven hammer blows.[5] But, as long as chiropractors applied the traditional medical dictum *primum non nocere* (first of all, do no harm), it would be difficult for them to lose.

Whether the healed patient decided to become a chiropractor or remained simply a lay advocate depended on the level of personal frustration and disappointment with the patient's lot in life. Early chiropractic bred true believers and helped satisfy what was essentially a religious yearning; a chiropractic career offered much more than simply an appeal to self-interest and a practical way for personal advancement. "Only a very few of the early chiropractors were young men seeking a prestigious way of making a living," chiropractor Walter Rhodes explained. "Most were appealed to by results they saw with their own eyes, and the logic of the explanations given for these results, which impressed them so much they desired to share it with all of humanity at whatever cost to the prestige they might already enjoy with their peers."[6]

Chiropractic did not develop as a practical organization, but instead bore the marks of a mass movement. Eric Hoffer has noted that a mass movement, "particularly in its active, revivalist phase, appeals not to those intent on bolstering and advancing a cherished self, but to those who crave to be rid of an unwanted self." The mass movement draws and retains its

CHIROPRACTORS HEAR WEBSTER BOY'S STORY OF SWALLOWED METAL

Ronald McCurdy Carried 2½-inch Piece of Metal in Body for 45 Days Before Elimination.

How a 2½-inch piece of metal lodged in a sac in a boy's intestines was removed by a basic technician was discussed as one of the most interesting cases of the year at the assembly of the chiropractors at the De Soto Hotel, June 22-26. This was the tenth annual assembly of the International Basic Technique Research Institute.

This technique was discovered and perfected by Dr. Hugh B. Logan. The boy whose body contained the elongated piece of metal for 45 days is Ronald McCurdy, 8, was was "eyed with awe" by his classmates in Webster Groves during the time he was a "guinea pig" while physicians studied X-rays. They gave up the idea of contact with instruments because the metal was too large to be brought back through the throat. He appeared at the Assembly in perfect health and described his painless recovery.

The mishap occurred to Ronald while he was lying on the floor of his room in the McCurdy home at 506 East Lockwood avenue, idly tossing the metal into the air as he listened to the radio. It dropped into his mouth, he gulped, then realized he had swallowed it. With his parents, Mr. and Mrs. Robert G. McCurdy, he made several trips to the hospital. As the metal began its journey through the stomach, at one time surgeons prepared to operate. It passed through the small intestine and became lodged at the caecum, the blind pouch or sac in which the large intestine begins.

Dr. A. L. Nickson, a basic technician and neighbor of the McCurdy's, had the boy sleeping at night and reclining at day in an almost "upside down" position. Then with the use of Basic Technique he was able to dislodge the metal from the sac which held it, get it into the large intestine, from where it completed its journey through Ronald's body. During all entire time the boy suffered no discomfort.

Piece of Metal Swallowed by Boy Slowly Passing Through Body

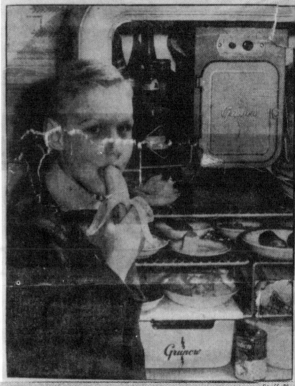

—Staff Pho

RONALD McCURDY,
who still has a man-sized appetite.

Ronald McCurdy, 8, is eyed with awe by his classmates at Holy Redeemer Parochial School, Webster Groves, because a piece of metal 2¼ inches long and a half inch wide is slowly working its way through his body, its course charted by physicians and surgeons, who study new X-rays every two or three days.

The boy was lying on the floor of his room in the McCurdy home at 505 East Lockwood avenue three weeks ago Sunday, idly tossing the metal into the air as he listened to the radio. It plopped into his mouth; he gulped in surprise, and then realized he had swallowed it. He went downstairs and told his parents, Mr. and Mrs. Robert G. McCurdy, and they made the first of several trips to a hospital.

Physicians decided, Mrs. McCurdy said yesterday, that it would be useless to attempt to contact the metal with instruments, because was too large to be brought bac through the throat. They were su prised the boy had been able swallow the metal.

The metal began its journe through the stomach, and at o time surgeons prepared to opera but when the metal moved agai it was decided to wait to determi if there could be a natural elimi tion. It passed through the sma intestine and at present is lodg at the caecum, the blind pouch sac in which the large intestir begins.

The youth suffers no discomfo and is continuing his normal rou tine, save for numerous examina tions by doctors. Thus far, X-rays have been made. His class mates and nuns at school are say ing prayers daily for his prompt re covery.

Boy Who Swallowed Metal Piece Gets Holiday—It's Out

Ronald McCurdy, 8, is going to Forest Park Highlands today and take in every ride in the amusement park. The piece of metal 2½ inches long and ¼-inch wide which he swallowed accidentally at April 26, completed its journey through the boy's body yesterday. Until a week ago the metal had been lodged in the lad's caecum, the blind pouch or sac in which the large intestine begins. Then Dr. A. L. Nickson, a basic technician and neighbor of the McCurdy family, which lives at 505 East Lockwood avenue, began treating Ronald. The treatments ended with natural elimination.

Ronald's parents, Mr. and Mrs. Robert G. McCurdy, were overjoyed. The boy had spent three weeks in a hospital, and at one time doctors prepared to resort to surgery to remove the metal. Then it moved from the stomach, through the small intestine into the caecum, where it remained until Dr. Nickson began his treatments.

The boy suffered no discomfort during the 45 days the metal was in his body. He returned to school for two weeks late last month and passed his second-grade final examinations at Holy Redeemer Catholic School with a 91 average.

For the last week, however, Ronald had to sleep almost "upside down," his bed having been raised at the foot more than a foot. More than 40 X-rays were made of the metal in various stages of its journey.

Walter E. Tiemann Dies in Atlantic City

Walter E. Tiemann, 47, president of the Tiemann Hardware and Supply Company, 2647 Locust street, died yesterday in Atlantic City.

Physicians were surprised the boy had been able to swallow the metal. They said at that time it was useless to contact it with instruments because it was too large to be brought back through the throat.

BOY SWALLOWS BIG PIECE OF METAL, LIVES

Dr. A. L. Nickson of St. Louis, Mo., son of Mrs. A. J. Nickson, 327 Weston avenue, and an East High graduate, brought happiness to the parents of an eight year old boy he attended after the youngster had swallowed a piece of metal 2½ inches long and half an inch wide.

The following account of the case is from the St. Louis Daily Globe Democrat:

"Ronald McCurdy, 8, is going to Forest Park Highlands today and take in every ride in the amusement park. The piece of metal 2½ inches long and ¼-inch wide, which he swallowed accidentally last April 26, completed its journey thru the boy's body yesterday.

"Until a week ago the metal had been lodged in the lad's caecum, the blind pouch or sac in which the large intestine begins. Then Dr. A. L. Nickson, a basic technician and neighbor of the McCurdy family, which lives at 505 East Lockwood avenue, began treating Ronald. The treatments ended with natural elimination.

Parents Overjoyed

"Ronald's parents, Mr. and Mrs. Robert G. McCurdy, were overjoyed. The boy had spent three weeks in a hospital, and at one time doctors prepared to resort to surgery to remove the metal. Then it moved from the stomach, thru the small intestine into the caecum, where it remained until Dr. Nickson began his treatments.

"The boy suffered no discomfort during the 45 days the metal was in his body. He returned to school for two weeks late last month and passed his second-grade final examinations at Holy Redeemer Catholic school with a 91 average.

"For the last week, however, Ronald had to sleep almost 'upside down,' his bed having been raised at the foot more than a foot. More than 40 X-rays were made of the metal in various stages of its journey."

THE AURORA BEACON-NEWS, Sunday, June 28, 1942.

FIGURE 12. Newspaper accounts of Dr. A.L. Nickson's successful treatment of Ronald McCurdy, age 8, who swallowed a 2¼ by ¼-inch piece of metal in 1942. Courtesy of Logan College of Chiropractic Archives, Chesterfield, Missouri.

The Metal

following "not because it can satisfy the desire for self-advancement, but because it can satisfy the desire for self-renunciation." The frustrated can lose themselves by melting into a mass movement that empowers them. "For men to plunge headlong into an undertaking of vast change, they must be intensely discontented yet not destitute, and they must have the feeling that by the possession of some potent doctrine, infallible leader or some new technique they have access to a source of irresistible power." In addition, true believers need a grandiose view of future potential and must be entirely ignorant of the difficulties of their sweeping venture. "Experience," Hoffer concluded, "is a handicap."[7]

Chiropractic converts were assured a millennial future if they combined patience with effort. Howard Nutting encouraged his chiropractic colleagues to "keep bravely on until the flag of chiropractic is unfurled in every town and hamlet; on until every asylum for the insane, for the inebriate and for the feeble minded shall be without occupants, or until the penitentiaries and reformatories are deserted and their crumbling walls and rusted bolts stand only as silent testimonials to the success of chiropractic."[8] In 1908, Nutting reminded fellow members of the Universal Chiropractors Association to heed well the name of the group. It was not simply a state or national association, he told them in biblical imagery, but one that "covers the universe" which "must be sown with chiropractic seed." Do not expect immediate success, he warned, "perhaps only a little patch here is prepared and sown, and then another; soon dotted here and there may be an oasis in the desert of prejudice and envy. Gradually these fertile spots will enlarge until, in the distant future, there will be one vast expanse of golden grain, the result of YOUR effort."[9]

Chiropractic drew not the destitute but the discontented, who came with little experience in medical matters. Martha Metz, D.C., in her scrapbook-style history of chiropractic in Kansas, noted that most "who took up chiropractic did so at an older-than-usual age, having left other occupations, due to their physical breakdown. Quite a few had been school teachers, some lawyers or preachers, office workers, and even druggists, while some were farmers and housekeepers or wives of the men who changed their life work and also studied with them." Metz concluded that such maturity carried with it an independence of mind and a "willingness to withstand persecution that others might learn the truth of a new system of healing, which had already been demonstrated in their own lives. They could stand alone in their convictions, rather than conform to the crowd."[10] Independent convictions, of course, meant independent in relation to outside detractors. Within the chiropractic fraternity, the basic convictions were already established, provided upon confession. That converts came to chiropractic with newfound strength drawn from vivid healings after earlier careers left them unfulfilled meant formidable allegiance to the chiropractic idea. Chiropractic provided a way to change the world.

Nevertheless, the chiropractic temperament was not entirely uniform despite the common threads of experience that brought most into the movement. Chiropractic drew believers with similar yearnings but with at least two clearly distinguishable temperaments that determined how their allegiance to chiropractic would develop. The first type came with deep spiritual longings but no strongly fixed religious faith when first introduced to chiropractic. For this seeker, chiropractic became a substitute religion, supplying a comprehensive explanation of reality, complete in itself with claims of divine powers, suffering saints and martyrs, and sacred writings and utterances from prophets (the Palmers) who provided the ultimate source of authority—all wrapped in a millennial eschatology. These Palmerites learned the sacraments well. In a graduation address delivered at the Palmer School in December 1906, Shegetaro Morikubo pleaded with fellow graduates to retain the sanctity of Palmer teaching.

> The science that possesses THE knowledge of cause of disease, regardless of character, needs no adjuncts. Secondly, the salvation to the species of living things is a continuance of its purity. Grafting of one species to another may please the fantasy and whims of our lighter nature; but sublimity and beauty are productions of singleness and purity. The future growth of chiropractic depends upon the preservation of its original cleanliness. The sublime climax of this science will attain its glorious height and splendor only when its followers remain unsullied in their scientific thoughts and art of applying it—adjustments. . . . It is my duty to promote my moral and intellectual integrity, to be sincere in purpose, and have rectitude of character worthy of a lover and worshiper of Chiropractic.[11]

Uncritical fidelity was the preeminent virtue for the true Palmerite. In 1910, Mary Deneen charged her fellow chiropractic students to "cultivate Loyalty in our school and be a little more appreciative, for few of us realize what a privilege we have, to be able to be at the Fountain Head where we get pure, unadulterated Chiropractic teaching with Dr. Palmer at the helm." Get yourself straight when dissatisfaction arises, she advised in the chiropractic version of repentance, "go off to yourself; think things over; ask yourself some questions. Are you doing your best? Can you do more than you are doing? Have you done everything you ought to?" B.J. himself provided the model for such self-examination and selfless devotion to chiropractic. "To say that he [B.J.] is giving his life for the advancement of pure and unadulterated chiropractic is but telling the truth," another votary explained. "He performs daily a herculean task, beginning in the quiet hour of two a.m., in order to be talking to his silent partner, Innate Intelligence, to whom he is a willing listener and pupil. Might we not discover the secret of this in 'the quiet hour with Universal Intelligence'?"[12]

In contrast to those who developed into Palmerites (and perhaps subsequently substituted another as prophet), a second type came to the movement with an orthodox Christian faith already in place, without need for the Palmer pantheon. Chiropractic failed to develop into a full-blown religion because for many (perhaps a majority),[13] Palmer chiropractic philosophy was co-opted by Christian orthodoxy; chiropractic became the Christian approach to health. Christian chiropractors were unwilling to adopt the Palmer views as a religion *in toto* but were willing to accept them as *part* of their religion by turning the chiropractic outlook and terminology down orthodox streets. Reverend Samuel H. Weed, the Presbyterian minister credited with coining the word *chiropractic,* explained with tendentious logic to those assembled in 1913 for D.D. Palmer's memorial service how chiropractic converged with Christianity. The Bible, he believed, provided numerous illustrations of chiropractic. For example, the word "Innate" appears in the Epistle of James (1:21), Weed held, when the believer is invited to "receive with meekness the engrafted word, which is able to save your soul" (King James Version). In the American Revised Version, "engrafted word" is translated as "implanted word" and a marginal note alternates the word "inborn," which, according to Weed, derives from the same Latin word as "Innate." Lange's Critical Commentary actually translates it as "Innate," that "Divine Intelligence or influence," Weed concluded, "that turns on the machinery of our bodies and heals our diseases. The Bible says: Heals all our diseases." The chiropractor is "simply a coworker with God."

Weed also claimed that the word "adjustment" is used several times in the New Testament. For example, in 1 Peter 5:10: "But the God of all grace, who hath called us into his eternal glory by Christ Jesus, after that ye have suffered a while, make you perfect, establish, strengthen, settle you." The word translated "perfect" means "adjust" in the original Greek, he explained; the American Revised Version renders it as "restores." An adjustment is merely a restoration of vertebrae to proper position, and "settle you" means "place you on a firm foundation." By this reading "we have the promise made to the Christians that after they have suffered a little while . . . He himself shall adjust, establish, strengthen you and place you on a firm foundation. That is one of the grandest climaxes that I know of in the Bible or in any other work."[14]

For a health reform ideology to draw inspiration and reinforcement from Christianity is certainly nothing novel. Christian chiropractors were spiritual descendants of antebellum health reformers, extending antebellum perfectionist thinking into the twentieth century. At the Chiropractors'

Convention of the East in June 1924, W.W. Parker explained in perfection-ist terms the crucial role of chiropractic for the well-being of mankind.

[Chiropractic] is not trying to inject something into the human system but [is] trying to bring the human system to that degree of perfection designed by the Creator when man was made. . . . Just as moral sin [*sic*—mortal?] has crept into the world, so has disease crept in. Man has the power of his will to overcome moral sin but disease is harder to combat and through our method we intend to restore mankind to his natural good condition.

He noted further the "great similarity" between the "indispensable miracle of Chiropractic" and "the wonderful healings of Jesus Christ."[15]

It required little imagination to identify Palmer's Universal Intelligence as the Christian God and Innate Intelligence as the divine spark of God in humans. Healing resulting from the chiropractic adjustment became an exhilarating work of God's grace, the physical counterpart to the spiritual grace that saved souls. Repentance was simply "surrender-adjustment to Christ," noted H.L. McSherry in "A Christian Concept of Chiropractic Philosophy," and "ADJUSTMENT is the key and slogan for our recovery," the avenue for complete grace, both physical and spiritual. The chiropractor functions as the medical priest who facilitates physical restoration and is the instrument by which God accomplishes the physical redemption of humans. "I believe, as a chiropractor," McSherry proclaimed, "that God has called us to appropriate and apply His revealed wisdom contained in chiropractic to man's body; that it is the most practical and constructive treatment for the human body; it is most in harmony with God's Natural Law; and is an important part of the progressive unfolding of God's will for us."

McSherry, however, no doubt expressing the thoughts of scores of Christian chiropractors, was careful to give Christianity preeminence, to test chiropractic in the crucible of Christian doctrine. Chiropractic philosophy first attracted him "as a Christian", he explained, because of its similarity to Christian philosophy. Without a concerted *religious* attachment to the Palmers, it became much easier for the Christian chiropractor to stray from Palmer technique and view the work itself as a mechanical approach to health. "Chiropractic," McSherry avowed, "is purely a mechanical science that assists nature in curing disease and maintaining health through human engineering. It is not a religion," he emphasized in boldface print, probably to combat the approach of the Palmerites, "yet its philosophy resembles Christian theology." Recognition of a first cause of all things, a theocentric viewpoint, and a "withinness" in both teachings (Jesus taught that "the Kingdom of God is within you," while the Palmers taught that the cause of disease is within you) were similar. The clergyman and the chiropractor both strive to keep humans "in tune with the same Infinite Intelligence," and both make the same "simplified, unartificial, nonmonopolistic, and democratic appeal," offering a "natural method for natural people." Chiropractic was the God-given way to health that "not only [was] scientifically and spiritually right, but also should appeal to the intelligent Christian and religious specialist as being morally right," quite in contrast to medical philosophy, "which is materialistic, and sometimes even atheistic." Medicines used by doctors are poisons that often create "evil effects," McSherry warned, so dangerous that the word medicine might best be rendered " 'MED-I-SIN'—and sin in any form we are definitely against!"[16]

The association of chiropractic with Christianity made its appeal far broader and its claims more persuasive than it would have been standing alone with only the Palmers as the source of authority. B.J. himself had little use for orthodox Christian faith (he approved only of the Mormon Church, Christian Science, and the Emmanuel Movement among religious bodies because they healed the sick by the laying on of hands) and was at odds with the Ministerial Alliance of Davenport, especially during the second decade of the century. His brash appraisal of the Ten Commandments as negative psychology, implying that God's understanding was faulty, was unlikely to endear him to Christians.

> The Ten Commandments are presumed to encompass the Golden Rule; they are so broad and long that the latitude and longitude cover every human endeavor. Yet, they have failed. They are ten in number, nine are negative and only one remains positive. "Thou Shalt NOT—" do this or that. Tell a boy he must NOT and he WILL. Tell humanity they shall NOT and they will violate an oath to do it. Commandments were written to prevent doing the thing they fasten upon. The paradox! Who ever wrote the Commandments did not know psychology or he would have written them in positive and then they would have accomplished, at least, more than they do.[17]

B.J.'s hubris served only to offend the orthodox. For Christians involved in the movement as both patients and practitioners, chiropractic became the medical adjunct of Truth, easily grafted to standing Christian beliefs. Chiropractic enlarged and complemented the Truth but could never replace it. For them, *Christian* chiropractic was the only kind.

Undoubtedly, some came into the fold without deep spiritual yearnings, wearing their righteousness less conspicuously than others and being more interested in making a respectable living than in ushering in the millennium. Almost invisible, overshadowed by the rhetoric of colleagues, they were surely there even in the early days of chiropractic. Though uninterested in buttressing the truth of experience with received doctrine, these unassuming advocates could still find a place in chiropractic along with both their dominant missionary brethren and the few inevitable charlatans because chiropractic was, if anything, an uncloistered movement with arms open.

WHO WAS WELCOME

Still, the open arms of chiropractic embraced with discretion. Racial prejudice, mirroring biases in the larger society, tended to bar blacks from full participation in the movement. After black janitor Harvey Lillard's highly visible role as recipient of D.D. Palmer's famed "first adjustment," blacks became virtually invisible within chiropractic, both as patients and as practitioners. The experience of chiropractor A. Augustus Dye, a product of the Palmer School (1912) who treated a number of wealthy clients in Essex County homes and New Jersey shore resorts, illustrates how white practitioners gingerly cared for black patients. Dye's well-to-do patrons frequently had black servants who also needed adjustment. "Of course," Dye wrote, "you couldn't use your portable adjusting table for both blacks and whites—if you hoped to retain the white patients." Dye explained his ingenuity in treating Bob Johnson, a black chauffeur who worked for comedian and movie actor Arthur Byron: "Naturally, I could not adjust him at my office nor at Mr. Byron's home. So, I had Bob make a table out of two beer cases, on which I adjusted him in the garage. Bob, being an intelligent negro, constructed a very serviceable table out of those cases." Another wealthy Dye patient "had a valued old negro maid that was under adjustment for a long time in the servant's quarters, and the employer, also taking adjustments at home, bought a table specially for her maid's use."[18]

As recipients of such segregated and surreptitious treatment, it is hardly surprising that few blacks rushed to become practitioners.[19] Those who tried found a color line encircling most chiropractic institutions. The "Fountainhead" Palmer School led the way by not admitting blacks; in the midteens its catalogue officially banned them from instruction ("with one exception," the copy read coyly, "its doors are open to all races"). In 1944, the policy was tested openly when B.J. reluctantly put the admission of black applicant Dorothy Clark to a vote at a student assembly after an alumnus agitated repeatedly for her acceptance. A majority bloc of southern students voted to leave school if the policy was reversed, and the ban remained in force for another decade. The threat of mass white exodus usually overcame any latent racial scruples, and most chiropractic schools, also proprietary, followed the Palmer policy, prohibiting black enrollment through the first half of the century.

Despite these widespread restrictions, some blacks still managed to find a way into the vocation. Some light-skinned blacks "passed" as white and enrolled in restricted schools, others kept their color secret by taking a D.C. diploma through correspondence schools, and others gained admittance to the few northeastern and upper midwestern schools that accepted black students. After World War II, black veterans with educational benefits from the G.I. Bill prompted the desegregation of some struggling chiropractic schools—a majority of black chiropractic graduates from 1949 to 1953 were veterans who used federal dollars from the G.I. Bill for chiropractic education. The G.I. Bill also created opportunities for aspiring educators as well as for potential black students. Booker T. Washington Chiropractic College (Kansas City, Missouri), International College of Chiropractic (Dayton, Ohio), and Bebout College of Chiropractic (Indianapolis, Indiana) all began operation in the immediate postwar era, graduating black chiropractors. After the July 1, 1951, application deadline for veterans' educational benefits passed, however, both Booker T. Washington and International soon closed, suggesting a close link between the G.I. Bill and the survival of schools that catered to black veterans.[20]

Although the economics of the G.I. Bill served to reduce overt racism in chiropractic, subtle *sub rosa* discrimination persisted, ranging from the failure of school clinic directors to assign white patients to black student doctors to unstated racial quotas at chiropractic colleges. Continued perception of discriminatory practices eventually induced chiropractor James Lavender, New Jersey Chiropractic Civil Rights Chairman since 1950, to submit a formal charge of discrimination in 1967 against Palmer College under Title VII of the 1964 Civil Rights Act. Lavender's request that federal funds be denied to schools with restrictive practices remains on file. In 1979, the National Association of Black Chiropractors and Community Development Volunteers filed charges of discrimination and de facto segregation against the Council on Chiropractic Education and a number of chiropractic colleges. In response, the Office of Civil Rights issued mild "letters of finding" to the colleges implicated, recommending revisions in catalogues and admission forms.[21]

Although formal charges seemed to accomplish little of substance, the issues raised by the complaints heightened sensitivity for black rights within chiropractic. Still, the black presence within the profession as well as awareness of chiropractic in the black community has remained minimal. By 1978, approximately 1 percent of American chiropractors and students were black, a percentage that endures. A survey of four chiropractic colleges in the mideighties revealed only seventeen black students in a combined student enrollment of 1,894, just under 1 percent. In St. Louis (where 9 of more than 600 practicing chiropractors were black), a sampling of inner city, black residents in the early eighties indicated that, although 78 percent had experienced back trouble, only 1 percent had received chiropractic treatment. By the late eighties, only 200 of some thirty thousand American chiropractors were black.[22]

In sharp contrast to the black experience in chiropractic, women established a significant presence, especially in the early years. Of the first "Fifteen Disciples" of D.D. Palmer's Chiropractic School and Cure (those who graduated before B.J. took his diploma in 1902), three were women and one, Minora Paxson, co-authored the first textbook of the profession and was probably the first chiropractor to pass a state board (under Illinois' "Other Practitioner" statute). Almeda Haldeman, a 1905 graduate of a Palmer offshoot school in Minneapolis also known as the Chiropractic School and Cure, became Canada's first practicing chiropractor after establishing a homestead in Herbert, Saskatchewan.[23]

Women spearheaded other chiropractic firsts and continued to be highly visible. In early May 1915, Kansas governor Arthur Capper appointed Anna Foy and Mrs. H.A. Post along with three men to administer the nation's first chiropractic law passed two years earlier. In recognition of faithful service to the cause, board members chose Foy as first president (a title she eventually held for twelve of the twenty-seven years she served) and on May 12, 1915, awarded her state license number 1. The percentage of women on this first board held for the state at large. By 1925, 40 percent of the state's recorded chiropractors (210 of 525) were women.[24]

In some areas, the ratio of women to men could occasionally range even higher than in Kansas. City directories of Washington, D.C., for 1913 and 1914 show that five of the ten District chiropractors were women and, in 1919, sixteen of thirty-three. By 1921, the ratio slipped to thirty of ninety-two,[25] a figure more typical for the profession nationwide. Scattered evidence from class and group photographs, state convention snapshots, and commencement announcements from the first three decades of chiropractic indicates that one-fourth to one-third of its practitioners were women, a figure significantly above that of orthodox medicine for the same period.[26]

Irregular medical sects have tended to attract more female practitioners than has regular medicine, but even among the unorthodox early chiropractic seems to have outstripped its predecessors.[27] Chiropractic may have held a special attraction for women, as both practitioners and patients, because it promised to eradicate disease by restoring proper nerve flow through natural means at a time when common wisdom charged women with particular susceptibility to nerve weakness or "neurasthenia," the catch-all calamity that New York physician George Beard had diagnosed as peculiar to modern civilization. The spine itself, the focus of chiropractic attention and the primary conduit of nerve flow, had long stood as a special symbol of the state of women's health. Dioclesian Lewis, foremost advocate of the "New Gymnastics" that swept the nation in the 1860s and beyond, had argued that the primary question a young woman should be asked upon entering school was not "how have you progressed in latin, but 'Miss

Mary, how is your spine?' "[28] Common knowledge also invested women with a natural gift for nurturing and healing the afflicted; few would have argued with educator Ella Flagg Young's observation that "every woman is born a doctor," but "men have to study to become one."[29]

Chiropractic offered a logical outlet for feminine curative powers, combining nature and nerves in a way that would make special sense to women. That many also believed women incapable of scientific rigor was no major hindrance (as it became to women who attempted to practice within the rising standards of scientific objectivity and rationality in orthodox medicine) in a field where empiricism continued to outrun theory. In chiropractic, women could continue to nurture the traditional virtues of gender—the personal, natural touch—that appeared increasingly irrelevant for modern medicine. Sometimes those virtues combined with others far less esoteric. Bronx chiropractor Anna Monteforte explained with the practical inclination and disarming simplicity often typical of chiropractors how women held a physical advantage even within her profession: "I believe that as a rule women have softer, more flexible hands than men, and this gives them a decided advantage in the field of chiropractic." Monteforte also expressed the traditional ideas of gender and illustrated how easily a commonplace notion can be translated into "fact": "It has often been said that a women's intuition is very strong and I believe this fact aids them in understanding their patients far better than a man would."[30]

In addition to any physical or natural disposition that induced women into chiropractic, many who otherwise may never have become practitioners entered the profession as helpmeets to their husbands, encouraged to matriculate by tuition breaks offered for spouses. Mae Parsons, for example, explained that she entered chiropractic with her husband in the second decade of the century not "seriously intend[ing] to practice . . . [but] became greatly interested."[31] After graduation, husband and wife usually practiced as a team, sharing a sense of equality and often a special comradery. Arthur and Vi Nickson described their joint practice, which began in the late thirties, as a "tag team" that worked together smoothly. In their lean, early years, Vi would often slip out of the office while the all too infrequent patient waited for treatment. She then phoned Arthur several times within earshot of the patient first to cancel and then to make fictitious appointments to explain the empty waiting room and to create an illusion of prosperity. Still, despite shared ruses and joint practices, women who worked with husbands were less than independent, autonomous practitioners. It was Vi who assumed responsibility for office details, answering the telephone and recording legitimate appointments while Arthur adjusted the few patients who appeared for treatment.[32] Vi (and the women partners of husband and wife teams) assumed a role that illustrates subtle changes within the movement, changes that constricted both the number and role of women in chiropractic.

The Kansas Chiropractic Association, bastion for the significant involvement of women chiropractors, organized a woman's auxiliary for the first time in 1935.[33] The very existence of the organization indicated that women were moving from the role of primary healer to that of support for chiropractic husbands. The strong, independent female practitioner was becoming an anachronism and perhaps something of an embarrassment for chiropractic men who battled constantly to upgrade the public image of their profession. An official, two-page sketch of the history of Logan College of Chiropractic (Chesterfield, Missouri) described a new course that clarified, in retrospect, the proper place of women in the field after 1940. "A one-year course for chiropractic office assistants was begun in 1940," the outline noted with unintended irony, "when the need became apparent for specially trained young women to assist the busy doctor of chiropractic. The demand for these young women assistants far exceeded the supply."[34] Women were to become subordinate assistants to bustling male chiropractors, replicating the role of nurses within orthodox medicine. Before long, "bring your wife" would become a typical postscript printed on invitations to chiropractic functions. Domesticity had come belatedly to chiropractic.

The shifting role of women in chiropractic was delayed temporarily during the war when the future of the profession itself seemed in jeopardy. Because chiropractic was excluded from the list of essential wartime occupations, both practicing male chiropractors and students were subject to induction. The draft seriously depleted the chiropractic ranks, and during the war years women constituted a large percentage of the severely dwindling numbers who studied chiropractic. Chiropractic functionaries, however, did not view a new influx of women into their schools as a potential solution. A National Chiropractic Association brief to the War Manpower Commission in March 1943 made it clear in a backhanded way that the future health of the profession depended on male students. Ominously, the report announced an impending shortage of qualified chiropractors and argued that "the exclusion of chiropractic from the list of essential occupations and the refusal to postpone induction of its students will, in the course of a few years, result in the extinction of the profession." Of twelve association-approved colleges, six had closed as aggregate enrollment slipped more than 50 percent, from 840 students in September 1940 to 404 in September 1942. The brief reported a recent census that revealed chiropractic as an aging profession with a declining number of women entering as practitioners. Of the 19,860 American chiropractors, 14,995 or 75.5 percent were forty-six or older; 25.3 percent were women. Only 4,865 practitioners were between eighteen and forty-five years old; just 15 percent of these (731) were women. The future vibrancy of chiropractic was tied to young men—without them, it seemed certain, chiropractic would wither. After studying demographic figures reported in the April 1943 issue of the National Chiropractic Association *Journal*, chiropractor W.T. Brown advised a fellow D.C. to "do a little calculating and WEEP."[35]

Ironically, the very war that threatened chiropractic also provided new life. Educational benefits from the G.I. Bill sent young veterans searching for a career, and many settled upon chiropractic. Men dominated postwar classes as enrollment surged; Rosie the chiropractor went home. Logan College, a representative institution that survived during the war years, graduated just thirty-six students from 1943 to 1945, but twenty-two were women. In 1949, only three women graduated among ninety. In the fifties, sixties, and early seventies no more than four women ever graduated with any class—in some years no women at all took a diploma. Women now trumpeted the cause primarily as patients and "posture queens" (fig. 13) rather than as practitioners.[36]

Only within the past fifteen years has the percentage of women chiropractors begun to rise, emulating the trend for women in other professions. By 1982, female students totaled 18 percent of national chiropractic enrollment, rising to 22 percent by 1985. From 1982 to 1985, women chiropractors increased from 6 to 8 percent of the profession (about half the percentage of female doctors in regular medicine), and by mid-1986 the figure had risen to 10 percent. In 1985, the International Network of Women Chiropractors organized with the express purpose of addressing the needs of women chiropractors from a feminist perspective and seemed to assure that women's voices would again be heard within the profession. After a hiatus of almost three decades, women were back and seemed targeted to regain a semblance of their former presence within the profession.[37]

MAKING CHIROPRACTORS

Whether black or white, male or female, inspired by millennial hopes or interested simply in a livelihood, all aspiring chiropractors entered the field through some manner of training. Early diplomas from Palmer's Chiropractic School and Cure proclaimed recipients as "competent" both "to TEACH and PRACTICE the same," opening the floodgates for informal apprenticeships and sundry schools. By February 1908, D.D. Palmer himself recognized the problems of such casualness. In a lecture in Oklahoma City, he lamented "that when I teach the science to one person and that person teaches it to another and the third person teach [*sic*] it to a fourth, that they get away from chiropractic until chiropractic in the hands of the third or fourth person is hardly recognizable as chiropractic."[38]

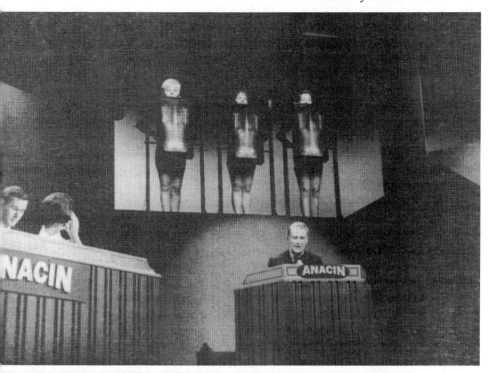

FIGURE 13. 1961 World Posture Queen Martha Jean Maxwell (on right) attempts to fool judges (including Johnny Carson) on "To Tell the Truth." From the *Digest of Chiropractic Economics,* January/February 1962.

The gradual development of more formal classroom instruction only multiplied the varieties of chiropractic. "Our schools," noted John J. Nugent, chief advocate for chiropractic educational reform, "presented a museum of diversity—a conglomeration of ideas, practices and prejudices as diversified as the individuals who controlled their destinies." As proprietary ventures, chiropractic schools had to consider the bottom line as carefully as any ideological purity. B.J. Palmer (who once commented unabashedly that his school operated on "a business . . . not a professional basis" and "manufacture[d] chiropractors") could wax indignant at the dishonorable motives of fellow chiropractic schoolmen. "The curse of Chiropractic," he charged, "is the army of scholastic pretenders, who, leech-like, have fastened themselves to the pedagogical phase of the vocation for the money there is in it." Many of these "scholastic pretenders" in turn denounced B.J.'s pecuniary motives, providing ample illustration from all sides of how a righteous sense of mission can easily obscure any lust for gain.[39]

With some 350 chiropractic schools operating sporadically within the past century, a certain number of pedagogical leeches was perhaps inevitable. In the teens, the American University of Chicago advertised its correspondence course in a variety of popular publications.

> BE A DOCTOR OF CHIROPRACTIC. Learn at Home in Spare Time. $3000 to $5000 a Year. The success of Chiropractors in many cases has come so quickly as to be almost startling. . . . NOW—Your Great Opportunity. . . . If you are ambitious to make money, increase your social standing and be "somebody," our course in Chiropractic will point the way. No special preliminary study required. You graduate with the degree D.C. (Doctor of Chiropractic), receive handsome diploma, FREE, and are ready at once to open your office.

If an inquirer returned the attached coupon, the university would rush twenty-two "magnificent charts" of the human body ("handsomely lithographed in life-like colors"—a regular $31.50 value) that showed how spinal pressure affected the various organs, along with an illustrated, seventy-two-page book and the particulars of the course, all without cost or obligation.[40]

In early 1915, George Creel targeted the American University for special censure in a series of exposés for *Harper's Weekly* on suspect medical practices. Creel quoted the form letter he received from "Dr. D.E. Wood, Dean," after responding to the school's ad. "Dear Friend" it opened, "If ever a note of inquiry was timely, yours is, . . . because right now there is a splendid opening for a doctor of chiropractic in your immediate vicinity, and nothing would please me more than to see you step in and fill it." The letter emphasized the ease of acquiring a diploma, leading to the "limitless field for legitimate big money making which this wonderful Science opens up!" The special offer of $68.75 for the complete course (payable in easy installments) was limited "strictly" to thirty days. When Creel visited the school's boiler room office on South Dearborn Street two months later, the literature packet he received addressed the same "Dear Friend" and made the same "strictly limited" offer.[41]

Such mail-order enterprises and subsequent exposés cast aspersions on all chiropractic schooling, yet the line between legitimate and illegitimate operations *was* often fuzzy for an aspiring profession prone to cure-all claims and unsure of its educational needs. Even the Fountainhead Palmer School briefly operated an adjunct School of Correspondence, and the National School in Chicago, considered by many to provide the best chiropractic education available, offered extension courses in ads similar to those of the American University, which only clouded the boundaries of legitimacy. The National School placed "The Grand Success of Chiropractic—An Unusual Opportunity" in the November 1913 *Cosmopolitan,* proclaiming chiropractic as "YOUR Opportunity." The ad invited the reader's introspection: "Are you ambitious? Do you feel that your abilities are fettered through circumstance—that you are fitted for something better in life than the position you occupy? . . . Why don't *you,* then, learn Chiropractic and become a personage of greater consequence, both financially and socially, in *your* community?" The science could be learned easily in spare time at home and in extension classes. A common school education would suffice to set the student on course for "rapid progress assured by fourteen big charts, including a life-span representation of the human body, drawn from life by X-Ray machine." All charts and a spinal column were promised "free" with the forty-dollar, fifty-four-lesson course.[42]

Although Abraham Flexner's famous 1910 report on medical education dismissed chiropractic out of hand as unworthy of consideration, subsequent medical writers such as Creel who took notice of the growing occupation made no real distinctions among the smorgasbord of chiropractic schools and courses but judged the field by the least worthy. A perennial tactic involved submission to chiropractic schools of semiliterate letters of inquiry that set forth less than impressive credentials. Responses from schools accepting these fictitious students were then published as evidence of nonexistent standards within chiropractic. The March 10, 1923, issue of the *Journal of the American Medical Association (JAMA)* reprinted *verbatim et literatim* one such letter, sent ostensibly by a twenty-four-year-old Texas widow, which used both money and good looks to bait the unwary proprietors of the Carver Chiropractic College of Oklahoma City.

> Sirs, Mister Kirpatic School. I want to rite letter an see if i can be kirpatic dr. if you can make a kirpatic dr. for how much money i got about 2 thousend dolers that my husband got wen he died from the insurance company that paid 3 thousand dolers but I had ode lots of money and funerl an everything cost more 1 thousand dolers. Could i be kirpatic dr. for this much money about 2 thousand dolers in bank. i been nurse some and help drs. and kirpatic dr say i am strong and pretty an i make good kirpatic dr. since my husband die I can live with my ant here in [town name omitted by editors] but it is my money in bank. My ant say i have not been in school enuff but my father live on ranch an work wen I was girl and I go to school 3 years. My husband die with apensitis in his side an drs. say it to late after they operate an lots of pus an kirpatic dr. say he could cure him if i had called him but i did not no it that is why i did not send for him an i want to be kirpatic dr so i can cure apensitis sometime. I been ritin some other kirpatic schools and kirpatic colleges but they send me books and dont anser my letters so i can no. if you will anser my letter an tell me if you can make me a kirpatic dr. on how much money i got an how long it will be if i am a widow 24 years old and i will come right away.

The editors of *JAMA* also reproduced the school's response, which consoled the grieving widow and commended her faith in chiropractic and her resolve to spend the money in preparing "for a real life's work." Lack of education should not cause her undue concern, the letter noted in a run-on sentence that rivaled some penned by the "widow": "While your education may be limited you have the intelligence and the determination and sufficient education to understand the English language you would have no difficulty in getting a knowledge of this subject so that you could go out and practice and be efficient." She was then offered immediate admittance; graduation would come in eighteen months "upon making your grades."[43]

In some quarters, chiropractic education indeed seemed a contradiction in terms and making the grade was less than arduous, but many chiropractors distanced themselves from the inferior schools and demanded that proper distinctions be drawn between true chiropractors and those who only traded under the name.[44] By the midteens, a number of chiropractic schools were expanding curriculum and lengthening course time in an attempt to upgrade the profession. Elevation of educational standards became a bootstrap operation and in many ways replicated the evolution of regular medical schooling during the nineteenth and early twentieth centuries. As with early chiropractic schools, American medical schools traditionally had emphasized practical education in proprietary schools with short, vocational terms where the faculty consisted of practitioners who taught only part time. Medical schools also advertised for students and frequently appealed to restless adults seeking a second vocation. By the late nineteenth century, medical education was mired in a proprietary tradition that accepted most comers. As late as 1887, an eight-year-old girl who applied in her own handwriting to a host of medical schools was accepted at more than half of them even though she stated clearly that she met none of the admission requirements. By 1900, 151 medical schools competed for applicants (some four hundred schools had been founded in the course of the previous century); higher standards only translated into fewer students and reduced income. Attempts to upgrade the profession served instead to undermine it.[45] This same dilemma faced chiropractic.

The transformation of regular medicine in the early twentieth century consisted mainly in raising the training and status of middling doctors and eliminating the bottom entirely, rather than elevating the status of those at the top.[46] Abraham Flexner had persuaded the Rockefeller family to grant an eventual sum of almost fifty million dollars to the medical schools he had judged worthy. Rockefeller money, along with funds from other philanthropists, broadened the gap between the better and poorer schools, dooming the latter to extinction. By the midtwenties, endowment income had become the second largest source of funds for medical colleges and meant the difference between making it as a class "A" institution or closing their doors. By 1930, the number of American medical schools had dropped to sixty-six.[47]

The transformation of chiropractic also depended primarily on eliminating the bottom of the profession; ultimately, survival would be tied to the viability of its schools. No chiropractic Rockefeller, however, emerged to ease the transition. Without foundation largesse, the inverse relationship between students and standards continued to stymie any attempt to reform education and eradicate the underside. Despite the apparently sincere motives of most who entered the field, chiropractic spawned its share of money-grubbers and hustlers who hindered reform. Chiropractor G.W. Hardie, a 1915 Palmer graduate, analyzed these base elements in a July 23, 1923, response to a prospective student who had written him for advice on whether to take up study.

> The average product turned out, or rather those run through those [chiropractic] diploma mills, have little ethical feeling. Their god is the dollar. They are cutting each other's throat for patients. Selling adjustments for a quarter and some less than that to those who want cheap adjustments. In almost every community some "nut" thinks he is divinely inspired and starts a school of his own. He teaches two hours three evenings a week and at the end of six months gives his dupes a diploma so large it could be read from an aeroplane. The statistics compiled by one of the largest schools in existence show that seventy per cent of the graduates of their institution failed to establish practices that kept them in the profession.

Still, Hardie saw a vast field of opportunity for a man "more interested in human welfare than in dollars" and encouraged his correspondent to look over the various schools carefully before matriculating.[48]

The worst educational offenders were ultimately self-defeating; woefully deficient education combined with mercenary motives meant that many graduates of diploma mills were unable to sustain a practice. By 1925, sixty-seven chiropractic schools had folded, while sixty-five continued in business.[49] Although this meant that an ample number of suspect operations and ill-trained practitioners continued to hinder the profession, a chiropractic Darwinism and gradually rising standards designed to meet newly implemented state licensing laws were beginning to accomplish for chiropractic what foundation grants had achieved for the medical profession.

In the midthirties John J. Nugent (1891–1979), described aptly by one observer as chiropractic's Abraham Flexner, vigorously attacked inferior schools still immune to tooth and claw. An Irish-born graduate of the National University of Dublin, Nugent emigrated to the United States in 1914. After appointment to the special Officers Candidate School at West Point and subsequent wartime duty, he rejected an offer to study at Yale

Law School and enrolled at the Palmer School in August 1921. His days in Davenport were stormy. President B.J. Palmer expelled him in June 1922 for "disloyalty, disrespect and insult to the President and circulating statements derogatory to the welfare of the institution." Exactly what Nugent did remains a mystery, but it certainly involved severe disagreement over educational standards. A faculty vote reinstated him in July, and Nugent soon graduated, while his enmity against B.J. intensified. In later years, as Nugent championed the reformation of chiropractic education, B.J. scorned his plans as "Nugentism" and branded him "the Antichrist of Chiropractic."[50]

What "Nugentism" meant began evolving when Nugent spearheaded the formation of the National Council on Chiropractic Examining Boards in 1935, the first effective committee on standards within the profession. After personally inspecting each of the thirty-seven remaining chiropractic colleges over the next few years, Nugent recommended the establishment of an educational code, the first step toward accreditation of chiropractic institutions. In 1939, the National Chiropractic Association (NCA) merged its newly formed Committee on Educational Standards with Nugent's council and named Nugent the NCA's first Director of Education, granting him authority to supervise accreditation based on his previous code.

Only twelve schools gained "provisional, approved ratings" from the committee in 1942 (a list that excluded the Palmer School); by 1946, closings and mergers helped reduce the number to only four. "Nugentism" cut a wide swath across both "straight" and "mixer" operations because, above all, it demanded the abolition of proprietary schools. In addition, Nugent's code mandated a high school diploma as the minimum preliminary education and insisted on a four-year course of chiropractic study ("four years of nine") that adhered to uniform standards approved by a professional accrediting agency. "I am the symbol of revolt against Palmer [fundamentalism] in this country," Nugent told an interviewer in 1949, "and I am hated by many in chiropractic for that." In defiance of Nugent's attempted reformation, B.J. retained Palmer's eighteen-month course until 1958, railed against higher educational standards at state chiropractic conventions, and frequently blasted Nugent's "Bluff and Hooey" from the pages of his *Fountain Head News*.[51]

B.J. was never convinced that any education beyond fundamental chiropractic training was either necessary or desirable for a chiropractor. B.J. was strongly against his son Dave's desire to attend college and, when Dave returned from the University of Pennsylvania's Wharton School of Finance and Commerce with degree in hand, B.J. cited his defiance and at first refused to let him in the house. It was Dave who would turn the Palmer School into an accredited nonprofit organization upon B.J.'s death in 1961.[52] From B.J.'s perspective, any type of accrediting was suspect because it diminished his power within the profession and tended to stifle his own chiropractic innovations. Earlier in the century, the inconsistent and highly fluid body of chiropractic knowledge, along with B.J.'s power of resistance, kept any move toward educational credentials at bay. As his influence waned, defying Nugent and circling the wagons with true Palmerites became his way of striking back at a profession that had relegated him to side stage.

But B.J.'s approach was anachronistic in an age enamored with credentials. It was Nugent, aided by rising postwar enrollments, who pointed the way to the future. He was the first to recommend at least two years or sixty semester hours of preprofessional college study for prospective students, a prescription adopted by the NCA's Council on Education in 1953 but rarely implemented in chiropractic schools until the sixties. In 1963, the NCA reorganized by merging with several smaller groups and formed the American Chiropractic Association (ACA). By this time, Nugent had retired and memory of his work had faded within chiropractic circles, but his basic vision of upgrading and standardizing the profession continued to guide the reformation. The ACA's Department of Education established standards for audits, finances, on-campus inspections, and evaluations. In 1974, the United States Office of Education recognized the ACA's Council on Chiropractic Education (CCE) as chiropractic's official accrediting agency. With licensure secured in all fifty states and chiropractic eligible for Medicare payments, an educational boom was on. Five new colleges soon opened (University of Pasadena College of Chiropractic, Pacific States Chiropractic College, Northern California Chiropractic College, Sherman College, and Life Chiropractic College), and a standard curriculum of 1,840 hours of basic sciences (anatomy, physiology, chemistry, pathology, hygiene, sanitation, and public health), 2,080 hours of clinical sciences (diagnosis, gynecology, obstetrics, pediatrics, roentgenology, geriatrics, dermatology, syphilology, toxicology, psychology, psychiatry, jurisprudence, ethics, economics, and principles of chiropractic), and 80 hours of electives soon became the norm.[53] The new-style missionaries of health went forth armed with impressive, standardized credentials that emulated those received by medical doctors. From the days when $500 and a few weeks of "training" or $68.75 and a stamp were enough to enter the field, chiropractic had traveled a long way.

Chapter Six

Bones of Contention: Vertebrae, Money, and Authority

Oh, you docs! . . . You're all alike, especially when you're just out of school and think you know it all. You can't see any good in chiropractic or electric belts or bonesetters or anything, because they take so many good dollars away from you.

Sinclair Lewis, *Arrowsmith*

I at first decided he [B.J. Palmer] was only a "common liar," but upon more mature deliberation I rather felt inclined to honor him with the more distinguished title of "an expert liar," but my conscience would not permit me to let him off so easy, for it was plain that he was a "damn liar." However, to give him all the credit due, I will just say he is "a common, expert, damned liar." As egotistic as a Chinese God and as ignorant as an African cannibal.

F.F. Farnsworth, M.D., *West Virginia Medical Journal*

The first medical society in Connecticut, organized in Litchfield in 1767, set the agenda for subsequent generations of doctors. Its purpose, according to an ex-member, was "to promote a good agreement, and harmony amongst its members, endeavour to be mutually assisting to each other, in the healing art, and to keep out all Quacks and vain pretenders to Physic. . . . The grand thing . . . is to keep out Quacks, and pretenders."[1]

This incessant contention in America between orthodox practitioners and "vain pretenders" has been a struggle primarily over authority and only secondarily over competition and money. In medical matters, money flows from authority and whoever establishes authority will ensure a steady flow of patients and dollars. Paul Starr distinguished *social* authority, which entails "the control of action through the giving of commands" (and therefore pertains only to social actors) from *cultural* authority, which involves "the construction of reality through definitions of fact and value" (and therefore may also dwell in cultural objects such as religious texts, dictionaries, or scientific works). Cultural authority, which became the basis of medical sovereignty, consists of two major components—dependence and legitimacy—and orthodox medicine had to establish both before their blasts against the unorthodox became convincing. At the end of the nineteenth century, widespread public acceptance of the complexity of the human body and its illnesses helped create psychological and emotional dependency as the sick surrendered private judgment to doctors who laid claim to understanding. The medical profession also generated dependency through various "gatekeeping" functions, determining, for example, who would enter hospitals and who would be reimbursed by insurance companies for medical expenditures. Legitimacy came through rising educational standards and strict licensing procedures, all based on a perceived equation of medicine with science. In the twentieth century, science became a word to conjure with and the medical profession developed as the scientific arbiter of the body whose collective decisions represented a "community of shared standards," based presumably on objective, rational thought and empirical evidence.[2]

By the time chiropractic became worthy of notice as a serious competitor for the health dollar in the second and third decades of the twentieth century, the orthodox profession was well on its way to establishing cultural hegemony over matters of health. Chiropractic represented a particularly egregious affront to medical authority because it apparently cured a variety of ailments that still baffled physicians and lured patients with theoretical claims that had not met the test of scientific validation. Merely to survive, any irregular medical group must, at the very least, create psychological and emotional dependency among its clients by getting them well; to flourish, it must create a measure of cultural authority, which also requires legitimacy. Chiropractic was able to survive by creating dependency, but until it could garner legitimacy—on grounds now determined by the medical profession—authority would fail to root and chiropractic would remain only a marginal profession. Licensing laws put chiropractic on the road to legitimacy, but many viewed these laws as simply a mechanism designed to proscribe chiropractors from broad medical practice. Escalating educational standards helped considerably, but until chiropractic could demonstrate some scientific validity based on the knowledge and methods of twentieth-century science, it would merely subsist as a discipline on the fringes.

Communicating judgments of "scientific validity" to a broad public is accomplished largely through the popular, periodical press. Popular magazines possess a considerable measure of cultural authority and become important arbiters of legitimacy, reflecting as well as shaping popular attitudes. The struggle for legitimacy meant that chiropractors also had to battle an unsavory image generated by the popular press. Popular magazines, spurred by a concerted war against "quackery" begun in earnest by AMA publicists and public health advocates in the 1920s, had consigned chiropractic to the medical outback. Until the 1950s the overwhelming majority of articles on the subject of chiropractic were decidedly negative, but thereafter the traditional pillory of chiropractic in the popular press was accompanied and eventually supplanted by articles favorable to the practice (see Appendix B).[3] A moderating tone and an increasing number of articles on chiropractic coincided with dramatically expanding circulation for popular magazines in the postwar era.[4] Even the *American Mercury*, no longer edited by chiropractic-basher H.L. Mencken, was willing to print a chiropractic apologia alongside a comdemnatory piece by a physician. Chiropractic enjoyed the patronage of millions of Americans, an editorial comment noted. "Clearly, it merits public discussion; to ignore it is to run counter to the traditions of vital American journalism."[5]

In the fifties, writers began to acknowledge that chiropractic had staying power and widespread appeal. They noticed that after more than a half century of incessant medical denunciation and legal harassment, chiropractic still existed and was indeed licensed in the vast majority of states. Even those who stopped short of endorsement held a grudging admiration for the sheer doggedness of chiropractic. If chiropractic was so ill-conceived and harmful, the writers suggested, then why did a growing number of people swear by it? By the 1950s, the longstanding patronage demanded explanation and writers began to imply self-serving motives behind medical opposition to chiropractic, the flickering of a postwar challenge to medical authority that would swell to full-blown therapeutic dissent in the holistic health movements of the sixties and seventies, which disputed medical sovereignty.[6] By the midseventies the popular press fully reflected this dissent, which questioned intrusive surgery and the need for drugs, by applauding chiropractic. For editors, it became financially unwise to continue running pieces that condemned chiropractic out of hand when it enjoyed a secure legal status and an apparently growing public acceptance. Vital American journalism still had to sell.

Before chiropractic could edge toward legitimacy on the turf of science and before the popular press would turn from enemy to ally, survival was aided by new patterns within the medical profession that gave chiropractors a geographical niche in the medical landscape. During the second decade of the century, the Flexner Report of 1910 helped accelerate the trend toward rising educational standards within medicine, resulting in the closing of medical schools judged as inferior. Educational costs edged upward, constricting matriculation to more affluent students. The supply of physicians began to plummet and specialization, no longer tainted with the stigma of quackery, captivated the medical profession as medical science parceled the body into its constituent parts. Successful specialists needed to practice in a highly populated area to ensure that enough people succumbed to the particular diseases they understood or suffered injury to the specific body parts they healed. This flow of new medical doctors into urban areas meant that many rural areas began to lose medical service. In the February 12, 1927, issue of the *Journal of the American Medical Association,* AMA President William Allen Pusey noted that the average age of rural doctors in the United States was more than fifty-two years and that the supply of doctors in average rural counties was diminishing significantly. By choosing from each state (excluding Rhode Island) twenty towns each with a population of one thousand or less and then comparing the 1914 and 1925 directories of the American Medical Association, he found that by the latter year physicians had disappeared from 310 of the 940 towns that had had physicians in 1914. Further study indicated that irregular practitioners tended to fill the geographical vacancies. Sixty-four rural counties (five counties each in Arkansas, Missouri, New Mexico, and Oregon and four or fewer counties in twenty other states) lured no medical graduates in the decade before 1925 while a total of 121 irregulars moved into them.[7] There was now minimal competition with medical doctors in these areas, and chiropractors, prominent among the irregulars, often became primary care-givers treating a broad range of ailments.

Yet chiropractic was not restricted to rural areas. A 1932 study by Louis Reed revealed that, in the four states he examined (Connecticut, Colorado, Florida, and Minnesota), a greater proportionate share of chiropractors than physicians practiced in large cities. In these states combined, 14 percent of the chiropractors and 18 percent of the physicians resided in towns with a population under 2,500 while 39 percent of the chiropractors compared to 26 percent of the physicians practiced in cities with more than 200,000 inhabitants. In Florida, however, chiropractors were concentrated in towns of medium size with relatively fewer chiropractors than physicians in the bigger cities. More recently, the December 1978 issue of *Family Health* noted that the "vast majority of chiropractors operate in offices on their own, more than half of them in towns with populations of 50,000 or less, where there is often no major hospital and where medical doctors are reluctant to set up shop."[8]

Chiropractic was not confined to rural or urban areas, however they may be defined, but spread throughout the country into communities of all sizes, challenging medical authority by offering a cheaper alternative and producing a curious kind of competition. Even though chiropractors seemed to compete more directly with physicians in urban areas, the competition was still indirect because most patients first sought cures from medical doctors before frequenting a chiropractor. Medical doctors lost few dollars directly from chiropractic competition. Chiropractors understood this clearly and delighted in tweaking physicians with reminders of medical ineffectiveness. "Physicians may call us ignoramuses, fakers, or just plain idiots," Lyndon Lee wrote to the editor of the *Bronx Home News*,

> but the hard, cold fact remains that patients in ever increasing numbers are placing themselves in the hands of Chiropractors. And in every case it is found that they do not come to a Chiropractor until first having been handled by one or more medical doctors. Might we suggest that with this advantage the physician can put the Chiropractor out of business in short order if he will just cure that patient? There will then be nothing for the Chiropractor to do. In other words the physician, by the simple expedient of being successful, can make the chiropractor unnecessary.[9]

Despite any medical shortcomings, chiropractors and other irregulars were far from replacing the orthodox. In 1932, the Committee on the Costs of Medical Care, a privately funded and independent body of physicians, economists, and public health specialists who published twenty-seven reports on medical care in America, provided the first dependable statistics on national health expenditures. While 29.8 cents of the "medical dollar" (totaling approximately $3.66 billion in 1929) went to private physicians, only 3.4 cents went to all "cultists," even less than the sum (4.2 cents) that went to "miscellaneous." If the average gross income of some sixteen thousand active chiropractors in 1929 was $4,200 (as indicated by a small number of the committee's community studies), then chiropractic revenue stood at $67.2 million or 54 percent of the $124.44 million spent on "cultists" in 1929.[10]

Although this was still a considerable figure and may have inflamed a chronic "pocketbookitis" among physicians, as chiropractors charged,[11] what infuriated physicians most were the sweeping claims that became the stock in trade of chiropractic and served to challenge medical authority. The *New York State Journal of Medicine* for January 1924 quoted with exasperation from a textbook published by the Palmer School in 1921, which claimed cures for ills ranging from corns and cancer to gonorrhea and gleet. "For ingrowing toe nails," the writer quoted the advice of the Palmer text, "adjust the last lumbar. Only last evening I relieved a bad case of ingrowing toe nails by one adjustment." And on hair: "I have on two occasions caused plenty of hair to grow on bald heads and two heads have changed grey hair to black by adjusting the 6th dorsal [vertebra] towards the right shoulder." These "hand magicians" perpetrated "foolish nonsense," the writer charged and then offered a diagnosis and prescription that became the standard medical incantation against chiropractic—it is "scientifically unsound and should be fought like a plague."[12]

No "hand magician" was likely to incite greater derision than B.J. Palmer, especially when he announced the "Hole-in-One" (H-I-O for short), a novel cervical adjustment technique that stirred a major controversy even within chiropractic. According to B.J., a great master at any task demonstrates proficiency by accomplishing his objective with as little effort as possible; a golfer's hole-in-one is the ultimate example. A chiropractor "may be in the Bobby Jones class and play in the '60's,' or he may belong to the 'tall sticks' and play 'Civil War golf'—out in 61 and back in 65. . . . Those who play the *'Hole In One'* game, whether it be golf, baseball, or *Chiropractic,* specialize and centralize their thot [*sic*], time, money, effort and ability." The master seeks to lower the score; the practitioner who plays "championship Chiropractic" will not waste time with "shot-gun" adjustments. *"The less you do, if done right,"* B.J. explained with emphasis, *"the greater will be the results. The more you do, if done wrong, the less will be the results."* There were both Bobby Joneses and Babe Ruths in chiropractic. The champion chiropractor will find the specific spot that needs "concentrated delivery" and "make a *'Hole In One'* or a *'home run'* to health."[13]

Such homespun logic struck physicians as simple-minded ignorance. B.J. agreed with them. "I hardly blame the physician when he calls the chiropractor ignorant," he proclaimed. "We *are* ignorant of everything *he* thinks essential. I call *him* ignorant. *He* is ignorant of everything I think necessary. . . . Because our problem and its solution is opposite, each thinks in terms of the opposite, acts in terms of the opposite, and accomplishes objectives in terms of the opposite. That is why he is a physician, and I am a chiropractor."[14] But B.J. was wrong in making his frequent assertion that medicine and chiropractic were opposites. Because the chiropractic art focused on Matter, particularly the vertebrae, its efficacy was potentially verifiable on scientific grounds. Christian Science, which concentrates exclusively on Spirit, and not chiropractic, stands in opposition to medicine.[15] As a pamphlet issued by the American Chiropractic Association in 1986 noted, "through basic research the validity of chiropractic theory can be tested, and through clinical research the effectiveness of chiropractic treatment can be evaluated."[16] Chiropractic and medicine could find common ground by battling over Matter, but modern science, already co-opted by medicine, set the agenda in this realm. To gain the final measure of legitimacy and with it the potential for cultural authority, chiropractic would need to prove itself by the standards of medical science, on the hustings of the medical profession.

SNAP, CRACKLE, AND POP: THE SCIENCE OF SPINAL MANIPULATION

Medicine may have co-opted science, but the association was far from giving doctors exclusive or complete knowledge over all systems of the body. "As incomprehensible as it may appear, the medical profession is woefully deficient in a knowledge of the spine and its importance in the treatment of disease," judged Alfred Walton, M.D., in a 1927 booklet. "Men of scholarly learning, and of true scientific discernment, have investigated with great patience almost every conceivable avenue of research bearing upon the cause of disease, but the importance of vertebral displacement, as a causative factor, has been ignored or greatly underestimated."[17] More recently, physician John McMillan Mennell, an expert on manipulative techniques, explained that the entire medical school curriculum is devoted to approximately 40 percent of the body and virtually ignores the musculoskeletal system, the other 60 percent.[18] Researchers have begun only lately to abandon polemics and consider seriously the biomechanics of spinal manipulation and its effects on health.

Spinal manipulation is a type of mobilization of the vertebrae, an assisted motion applied to the spinal process (the natural vertebral outgrowth) and to sacroiliac joints. Yet manipulation requires a skill that goes beyond mobilization. A synovial joint[19] has an active range of motion (ROM) and a small buffer zone of passive motion (fig. 14). Mobilization occurs when a joint is assisted into this passive range. An elastic barrier of resistance exists beyond the passive ROM which has a spring-like feel and helps to stabilize the joints. Actual manipulation occurs if the joints are forced beyond the elastic barrier and the articular surfaces suddenly separate with a cracking noise. This additional separation is known as the paraphysiological ROM and happens only after a sudden release of synovial gases in the joint, the "crack" or "pop" that physicists call cavitation. For thirty minutes after release of the gas, the resistance between the passive and paraphysiological zones is gone, resulting in additional joint space. The elastic barrier is reestablished as the synovial gases are absorbed, but during this period additional manipulation is somewhat dangerous. At any time, movement beyond the paraphysiological ROM damages the capsular ligaments and threatens anatomical integrity. Painless manipulation, therefore, requires considerable skill and experience.[20]

Precisely what effect spinal manipulation has on pain is still theoretical, but the Gate Theory, first proposed in 1965, offers a widely accepted explanation. According to the theory, a spinal gating mechanism exists

JOINT MOBILIZATION and MANIPULATION

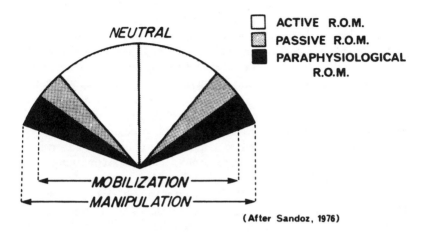

(After Sandoz, 1976)

FIGURE 14. Joint mobilization and manipulation. From W.H. Kirkaldy-Willis and J.D. Cassidy, "Spinal Manipulation in the Treatment of Low-Back Pain," *Canadian Family Physician* 31 (March 1985). Courtesy of W.H. Kirkaldy-Willis and J.D. Cassidy.

within the substantia gelatinosa (the substance that sheaths the posterior horn of the spinal cord and lines the central canal). This gating mechanism controls the transmission of sensory information such as pain, temperature, and touch. Research demonstrates that stimulation of bodily tissues can block the central transmission of pain, whereas lack of stimulation can facilitate pain—a concept that explains why rubbing an acute injury relieves pain and why early mobilization of a musculoskeletal injury can help control discomfort. The articular capsules of the spinal facet joints are heavily populated with sensitive nerve endings that relay information to the substantia gelatinosa through large myelinated fibers.[21] These impulses compete with smaller unmyelinated pain fibers from neighboring tissues for transmission. Stimulation that induces motion of the spine tends to decrease the transmission of pain from adjacent spinal structures by closing the gate. In this way, any therapy that creates articular motion will serve to inhibit pain.

No evidence exists to support the early chiropractic theory (which most present chiropractors have abandoned) that spinal manipulation replaces subluxated vertebrae. The old notion that a vertebra "went out," pressed upon a nerve, and then caused pain is the reverse of what appears to happen.[22] A *lack* of motion causes pain—a vertebra fails to move in one or more of its six normal ways. While offering suspect theory through the years, chiropractors have actually been restoring motion to inhibited joints. A new technique known as motion palpation, developed by a Belgian chiropractor and introduced in the United States during the fall of 1981, takes note of the gate theory and offers a diagnostic method of determining the specific failure of vertebral movement. From behind a seated patient, the chiropractor moves the patient's body with one hand while pressing on the vertebrae with the other. The areas of greatest immobility become the focus of manipulation. Success with manipulative therapy is greatest when the neurological deficit is not severe; manipulation of a prolapsed disc with extensive nerve damage, for example, would be contraindicated.[23]

That manipulation can provide relief from many musculoskeletal problems (known as type M disorders, such as simple backache or sciatica) is beyond reasonable doubt, but chiropractic claims that manipulation can also relieve organic or visceral disorders (known as type O problems, such as high blood pressure or diabetes) remain problematic. Traditionally, chiropractors have failed to distinguish between these two types of disorders, and their assertions that adjustments cure organic ills have especially raised the ire of the medical profession. Yet many patients have sought chiropractic relief from type M complaints and found to their (and often the practitioner's) surprise that a type O complaint was eased. To explain the result, chiropractors have theorized that spinal adjustment returns the body to more normal physiological functioning, enhancing the body's natural ability to deal with an organic disorder. Such a notion is extremely difficult to demonstrate scientifically and opens the door wide for the overzealous to claim cures for myriad ills. Discernment is complicated further by the phenomenon of referred pain—bodily pain that develops at a location distant from its cause. For example, a patient may have a vertebrogenic disorder that affects the adjacent nerves of the spine, but the resulting pain may appear in the chest rather than at the site of the dysfunction. This chest discomfort may mimic the pain associated with angina and may muddle correct diagnosis. The skilled chiropractor will find the vertebral problem and ease the pain, but if the patient receives no explanation of the phenomenon he might assume that the chiropractic treatment cured him of heart disease, a condition that may have been impervious to the ministrations of a medical doctor consulted previously. Conversely, an organic, viscerogenic disorder such as a digestive ailment can refer pain to the back and imitate the discomfort associated with a spinal problem. But these are merely simple examples. Pain can be referred from one part of the spinal column to another. Reflex sensory input from visceral sources can produce combined somatic and visceral effects, and sensory input from somatic sources can produce visceral and somatic effects in combination. Certain portions of the soma and viscera even share common segments of the spinal cord. In short, referred pain is deceptive.[24]

Understanding how this intricate web of nerves functions is a daunting task that requires painstaking research. Convincing theoretical explanations of chiropractic success have been especially difficult to generate because of a dearth of basic research by chiropractors themselves. The medical profession has offered meager help, since traditional chiropractic theories seemed so outlandish that physicians have been more content with polemics than with unbiased research. A major breakthrough for the scientific respectability of chiropractic came in 1974 when Congress appropriated two million dollars for the National Institute of Neurological Diseases and Stroke (NINDS) of the National Institutes of Health (NIH) to conduct an "independent, unbiased" study of the scientific basis of chiropractic. On February 2–4, 1975, NINDS convened fifty-eight scientists and clinicians (sixteen chiropractors, twenty-four medical doctors, seven osteopaths, and eleven basic scientists from the United States and eight foreign countries) at the NIH for a "Workshop on the Research Status of Spinal Manipulative Therapy." A shift in focus from the scientific base of chiropractic to spinal manipulative therapy broadened the investigation and helped steer attention away from longstanding medical and chiropractic rivalries. For the first time, chiropractors met with physicians and scientists on equal footing to consider an extensive agenda that included topics ranging from spinal geometry and kinematics to the pathophysiology of back pain. Although noting that specific conclusions either for or against spinal manipulative therapy could not be derived from the scientific literature and stopping short of endorsing the technique, the workshop refused to disqualify the subluxation hypothesis and called for additional experimental research.[25] That a prestigious international gathering treated spinal therapy respectfully and refused to dismiss it as quackery helped elevate the status of chiropractic. When "cranks" of any stripe promote a theory as scientific, the burden of proof—more aptly, the burden of disproof—lies primarily with skeptics rather than advocates; a theory will begin to dissolve when scoffers disprove it definitively. As long as a theory remains viable, especially one that yields beneficial practical applications such as chiropractic, it will persist. Refusal by the scientific community to dismiss is a major step toward acceptance and legitimacy.

Another major stride for chiropractic came from an unexpected source in January 1978, when Sir Keith Jacka Holyoake, Governor-General of New Zealand, charged a blue ribbon panel under the Commissions of Inquiry Act of 1908 to investigate and report upon the desirability of providing chiropractic benefits through the New Zealand Social Security

Act of 1964 and related aid under the Accident Compensation Act of 1972. The dimensions of the inquiry expanded rapidly and assumed implications for chiropractic far greater than simply the status of health benefits in New Zealand. The commission visited chiropractic colleges and held public sittings in the United Kingdom, Australia, Canada, and the United States while receiving 136 formal submissions of evidence from individuals and numerous medical and chiropractic associations. The findings soon developed into a referendum on chiropractic itself.[26]

Panel members admitted candidly in their report (running to 377 pages of text and appendices culled from thousands of typescript pages) that they began the inquiry with a vague impression of chiropractic as an unscientific cult, a notion they believed many in their community shared. Despite such an unpromising start for the fortunes of chiropractic, the panel concluded that modern chiropractic was far from being an unscientific cult, that chiropractors perform "spinal diagnosis and therapy at a sophisticated and refined level" and are the only health practitioners who are equipped by training to execute spinal manipulation. "By the end of the inquiry," the panel remarked,

> we found ourselves irresistibly and with complete unanimity drawn to the conclusion that modern chiropractic is a soundly-based and valuable branch of health care in a specialised area neglected by the medical profession. If properly controlled, it is worthy of public confidence and support. Health and accident compensation benefits should be made available, within the limits we define and discuss, for chiropractic treatment.[27]

Although acknowledging that precise scientific reasons why spinal therapy provided relief remained hazy, the commission was especially impressed with the clinical evidence for the efficacy of chiropractic. They recognized that experimentation in the laboratory provided only one method of validation. Clinical trial, the other tribunal of scientific medical practice, offered chiropractic a way of vindication which could move it beyond traditional reliance on anecdotal testimony.

CHIROPRACTIC IN THE CLINIC

Chiropractors, of course, have long made claims for clinical effectiveness; even when extending beyond the singular anecdote, however, their assertions were often statistically questionable and lacked the power to convince. A. Augustus Dye, an early, staunch advocate, simply asserted that from the "very start" of chiropractic, "practically 60% of the cases were partially restored to normal health with complete restoration in about 40% of the cases adjusted" and that, by the time he wrote, the percentage was "much greater."[28] After the flu epidemic that ravaged the nation throughout 1917 and 1918, Willard Carver reported that in Davenport, Iowa, 50 medical doctors treated 4,953 influenza patients with 274 deaths, while 150 chiropractors (including students and faculty at the Palmer School) treated 1,635 cases with just 1 death. He claimed that in New York City the epidemic took 950 of every 10,000 treated by medical methods, while only 25 of every 10,000 died under drugless care.[29] Given the self-limiting nature of the flu as well as possible cross treatments taken, concomitant illnesses, and a dearth of information on the age and general health of patients, such figures lack credibility.

To gain clinical credence, chiropractic would need more rigorous evaluation than that offered by anecdote or by self-congratulatory, intramural statistics. Since 1952, spinal manipulation for back pain has been tested in more than fifty clinical trials with at least a dozen both randomized and controlled. The cumulative trends indicate that, compared to other therapies, manipulation shortens the duration of pain in patients with both acute and chronic low-back ailments but fails to alter the recurrent nature of the problem. Initial improvement is followed by regression to the mean, yet this is also true with all other therapies. Even surgical intervention to repair a lumbar disc herniation (discectomy) eventually results in a similar regression.[30] A more recent, randomized British study, larger than previous clinical trials (involving 741 patients eighteen to sixty-five years old in eleven different English cities and towns) and with longer follow-up periods (lasting from March 1986 until March 1989), found chiropractic clinics more effective than medical clinics for low-back pain of mechanical origin, but contrary to previous studies discovered chiropractic results to be long lasting, especially among those who suffered severely upon entering the study or who had experienced previous episodes of back pain. Chiropractic seemed to have the *least* advantage over medical treatment for those who had no previous history of low-back pain. Although the long-term benefits of chiropractic remain an open issue, the studies indicate that, for low-back pain, chiropractic manipulation has the edge over medical management.[31]

Studies of workmen's compensation cases comparing medical and chiropractic care of back injuries have generally shown chiropractic to be more effective in reducing time lost as well as treatment and compensation costs. In March 1971, the medical director of the Workmen's Compensation Board of Oregon released "A Study of Time Loss Back Claims," an assessment of 237 claims for back injuries uncomplicated by attendant illnesses. Twenty-nine workmen were treated only by a chiropractor. Of these, 82 percent resumed work after one week without a disability award. Only 41 percent of the claimants treated solely by a medical doctor (with an injury judged comparable to those under chiropractic care) went back to work after one week.[32]

In 1972, physician C. Richard Wolf used records of the California Division of Labor Statistics and Research (Doctor's First Report of Work Injury) to compare medical and chiropractic treatment of industrial back injury. Wolf selected five hundred back injury reports signed by medical doctors and five hundred signed by chiropractors and sent questionnaires to each workman asking about time lost and residual pain. Wolf detailed the significant differences (see table 1). Befuddled by the results, Wolf could not explain the differences by any bias in the study design, "nor is there anything in the study to permit speculation as to relative treatment merits," he noted. "Therefore some explanation remains to come forth." Unable to offer one, Wolf simply concluded his report: "The author is unable to explain these differences."[33]

Explanations may have been lacking, but medical sources continued to document chiropractic effectiveness. The June 29, 1974, *Lancet* reported a survey of Utah state employees who had sustained work-related neck and back injuries between July and December 1972. Interviewers from the University of Utah College of Medicine questioned 122 chiropractic and 110 medical patients to determine their functional status before and after the incident and their satisfaction with the therapist and the care received. Surveyors found no statistically significant differences between the chiropractic and medical respondents regarding age, race, sex, educational background, marital status, income level, attitudes toward the medical profession, or hypochondria. Chiropractors required almost twice as many visits per patient compared to physicians (12.8 to 7.3), but the mean duration of chiropractic treatment was only 6.5 weeks measured against 9.3 weeks for medical patients. A sophisticated analysis of initial and final levels of functional status yielded no statistically significant difference between the groups of employees. The "ratio of improvement," however, indicated that physicians were "somewhat less effective" than chiropractors. Questions that measured patient satisfaction showed that a statistically significant proportion of chiropractic patients felt more welcomed than patients of physicians and were more satisfied with explanations of their problem and

TABLE 1 RESULTS OF MEDICAL AND CHIROPRACTIC TREATMENT OF
INDUSTRIAL BACK INJURY

Parameter	M.D.-treated Group	D.C.-treated Group
Average time lost per employee	32 days	15.6 days
Employees reporting no lost time	21%	47.9%
Employees reporting lost time in excess of 60 days	13.2%	6.7%
Employees reporting complete recovery	34.8%	51%

its treatment. The investigators concluded that, "although the theoretical basis of chiropractic is still unsubstantiated by traditional scientific evidence, none the less the intervention of a chiropractor in problems around neck and spine injuries was at least as effective as that of a physician, in terms of restoring the patient's function and satisfying the patient." They ended by recognizing the darkening "storm clouds" between the two professions and issued a call for "'definitive data" to replace "impassioned statements."[34]

Economic benefits have a way of eroding prejudice. Theory, after all, could wait. As studies mounted which indicated that chiropractic care could reduce cost and time lost over more traditional methods, health maintenance organizations (HMOs) and insurance companies began to take notice. Herbert H. Davis, M.D., Medical Director of AV-MED, the largest HMO in the southeastern United States, noted in a March 1983 letter to his chiropractic associates that the key to profitability for an HMO was cost containment rather than growth. Until AV-MED began using chiropractic services, he continued, they were spending "a considerable amount" on disc surgery and related problems. "Since I became enlightened about the benefits of chiropractic care," Davis wrote, "AV-MED's costs in this area have plummeted. Your conscientious approach in treating patients conservatively . . . has kept many useless hospitalizations and surgery [*sic*] from occurring." Davis then ended with a mea culpa: "I practiced medicine for twenty years and had certain prejudices about chiropractic care. You have certainly opened my eyes to its true merit."[35]

Davis had reason to rejoice. AV-MED's own "Study of the First 100 Patients Referred to the Silverman Chiropractic Center" showed that, before receiving chiropractic care,

—all but twenty patients had been treated by a medical doctor;
—the average patient had seen 1.6 doctors;
—seventeen had been diagnosed as having disc problems;
—four had received treatment in emergency rooms;
—two had been hospitalized;
—twelve had been diagnosed as needing surgery.

After chiropractic treatment, 86 percent did not need additional consultation with a physician and none of the twelve surgical candidates required an operation. AV-MED estimated that savings on the one hundred-patient sample ranged from $200,000 to $250,000. Davis was promoted from Medical Director to both President and Chairman of the Board.[36]

Clinical effectiveness helped to sustain and broaden the institutionalization of chiropractic. In 1974, Congress passed legislation providing for payment of chiropractic fees under Medicare. Such national recognition was augmented by three additional events of that year—passage of state licensing laws in Louisiana and Mississippi (the last two of the fifty states to license chiropractors), authorization by the United States Office of Education to the Chiropractic Commission on Education to begin accreditation of chiropractic colleges, and the congressional allocation of two million dollars to the National Institutes of Health for scientific study of the biomechanics of chiropractic manipulation. Nineteen seventy-four was the *annus mirabilis* of chiropractic.

By the mid-1980s, health insurance companies had also responded favorably to reports of chiropractic utility. Virtually every major commercial insurance carrier provided chiropractic benefits; more than three-fourths of the states required chiropractic inclusion in all commercial health-and-accident policies written within their borders. All fifty states, the District of Columbia, and the federal government had included chiropractic services within their workmen's compensation plans, and all citizens covered under Medicare, Medicaid, and the Vocational Rehabilitation Program were authorized to seek chiropractic treatment. Both the Railroad Retirement Act and the Longshoremen's and Harbor Workers' Act included chiropractic. The Department of Health and Human Services classified chiropractors as category 1 providers along with medical doctors, osteopaths, and dental surgeons. Even the niggardly Internal Revenue Service allowed the deduction of chiropractic costs as a medical expense.[37]

The demonstrated clinical successes of chiropractic coupled with plausible theoretical explanations moved chiropractic into the circle of legitimacy and smoothed the way for cultural authority over matters of the spine. This clinical success was communicated in the popular press, where chiropractors were beginning to emerge as back experts and the Horatio Alger heroes of the medical world. Since 1975, only two articles (both in *Consumer's Report*) still considered chiropractic to be a dubious method of healing.[38] *Prevention, Psychology Today, Sports Illustrated, Glamour, Good Housekeeping, Health, Esquire,* and *Mother Earth News,* among others, all reached millions with good news about chiropractic. The overwhelmingly positive message combined with the diversity and expanding circulation of publications printing chiropractic articles served to solidify chiropractors' therapeutic claims. The message was still frequently polemical, as it had been throughout the century, but the writers had traded sides in the course of the debate. Symbolic of the shift was the appearance of an article entitled "Chiropractic Comes of Age" in the December 1978 *Family Health,* a publication that recently had absorbed the AMA-published *Today's Health.* "Chiropractic works," *Family Health* quoted a plaque hanging in many chiropractic offices. "It gets results. That's what counts."

But chiropractic legitimacy had as much to do with politics as it did with science or public opinion and, until chiropractic could surmount the entrenched opposition of the AMA and its associated medical organizations, any authority would remain tenuous. After decades of securing sovereignty over the body, organized medicine was unwilling to relinquish even the vertebrae to chiropractic.

"Victory of the Century"

On October 1, 1976, Chester A. Wilk and four fellow chiropractors brought suit against the American Medical Association, the American Hospital Association, the American Academy of Orthopaedic Surgeons, five other medical associations, and four individuals, charging them with violating section 1 of the Sherman Antitrust Act by conspiring to eliminate chiropractic through refusal to associate professionally with chiropractors.[39] Section 1 of the Sherman Act prohibits agreements and combinations that improperly restrain interstate commerce or trade. In determining violations, the courts have used one of two approaches, the per se rule and the rule of reason. Under the per se rule, the court presumes that the defendant's conduct restrains competition unduly and may be condemned without an analysis of the effect or purpose of the restraint. The Supreme Court has ruled, for example, that group boycotts, horizontal market divisions, and price-fixing agreements constitute illegal per se arrangements. If the court decides that per se analysis is inappropriate, the rule of reason then applies. The purposes and probable effects of the defendant's actions are examined to determine whether or not they are anticompetitive. Typically, the defendant argues for the rule of reason; a strict per se analysis tilts the advantage to the plaintiff, since the plaintiff does not have to prove any actual effect of the challenged activity. In addition, under the per se rule the court considers irrelevant any justifications offered by the defendant for restraining trade. The plaintiff's chief hurdle in an antitrust suit is convincing the court to apply the per se approach rather than the rule of reason.[40]

The Wilk case first went to trial in Chicago on December 8, 1980, after four years of depositions. Attorneys for the plaintiffs sought to condemn the defendants' actions as a per se violation of the Sherman Act. Led by Judge Nicholas Bua's instructions implying that a "public interest motive" allows a defendant to escape the per se category, the jury found for the AMA. On appeal, Seventh Circuit Judge James E. Doyle ruled that, although the jury instructions were in error, any disadvantages to the plaintiffs were not prejudicial because the evidence of a "patient care motive" (a specific form of public interest) required a rule of reason rather than a per se analysis. Doyle then ordered a new trial under a "modified" rule of reason. The burden of persuasion would rest on Wilk to show that the primary effect of the defendants' conduct was to restrict competition. Defendants, in turn, would need to demonstrate a genuine concern for the scientific method in patient care and, if "objectively reasonable" as the dominant factor in their refusal to associate with chiropractors, that the concern could not have been satisfied in a less restrictive competitive manner.[41]

During the course of the trial, the plaintiffs presented evidence detailing the origin of an AMA plan to subdue and eliminate chiropractic. Plaintiff's exhibit number 172 shows that, in 1962, Robert B. Throckmorton, general counsel of the Iowa Medical Society (a constituent society of the defendant AMA), devised a plan to curb chiropractic in Iowa, a plan subsequently published for medical organization executives in November 1962 and read by Throckmorton at a Minneapolis medical conference in December. In a section entitled "What Medicine Should Do about the Chiropractic Menace," Throckmorton suggested that Medicine "encourage chiropractic disunity" and "undertake a positive program of 'containment.' If this program is successfully pursued," he continued, "it is entirely likely that chiropractic as a profession will 'wither on the vine' and the chiropractic menace will die a natural but somewhat undramatic death." He then outlined specific actions for pursuing the policy of "containment." Medicine should "encourage ethical complaints against chiropractors," "oppose chiropractic inroads" into health insurance, workmen's compensation, and labor unions, and "contain chiropractic schools." A successful containment policy "must necessarily be directed at the schools. To the extent that these financial problems continue to multiply, and to the extent that the schools are unsuccessful in their recruiting programs, the chiropractic menace of the future will be reduced and possibly eliminated." Section 3 of the document offered among its conclusions that "action taken by the medical profession should be . . . behind the scenes whenever possible" and warned physicians to "never give professional recognition to chiropractors."[42]

In 1963, the AMA officers invited Throckmorton to become their General Counsel and to initiate a medical unity campaign by implementing his Iowa plan of chiropractic containment on a national scale. On November 2 and 3, 1963, the AMA Board of Trustees voted to establish a "Committee on Quackery" (originally designated as the Committee on Chiropractic). The committee considered its "prime mission to be, first, the containment of chiropractic and ultimately, the elimination of chiropractic."[43]

Various AMA surveys between 1964 and 1966 indicating that physicians around the country were consulting with and referring to chiropractors alarmed the committee. In December 1966, the AMA House of Delegates, upon recommendation of the Committee on Quackery and the AMA Board of Trustees, adopted a resolution to ensure that all physicians understood clearly that principle 3 of the AMA's code of medical ethics, which forbade professional association with cultists and unscientific practitioners, applied to chiropractic. "It is the position of the medical profession," the policy stated, presuming to speak for all doctors, "that chiropractic is an unscientific cult whose practitioners lack the necessary training and background to diagnose and treat human disease." The AMA Judicial Council, often referred to as the Supreme Court of American Medicine, incorporated the policy into its Opinions and Reports, the official interpretation of the Principles of Medical Ethics. The Committee on Quackery viewed the policy as "the necessary tool" for widening the chiropractic campaign. "With it, other health-related groups were asked and did adopt . . . it," the committee noted. "These, in turn, led to even wider acceptance of the AMA position. . . . The hoped-for effect of this widened base of support was and is to minimize the chiropractic argument that the campaign is simply one of economics, dictated and manipulated by the AMA."[44]

The AMA's Department of Investigation, a clearinghouse for information on "unscientific" healing methods, combined with the Committee on Quackery to prepare and distribute to physicians and laymen a variety of publications critical of chiropractic. The committee actively discouraged colleges, universities, and faculties from cooperating with chiropractic schools and sent letters warning medical associations and boards that collaboration with chiropractors was unethical. State and county medical societies and individual doctors across the country became fearful that any contact with a chiropractor might taint them irrevocably. Physicians actually wrote to the AMA asking whether or not they would have to resign from Rotary Clubs and other civic organizations because chiropractors had joined. On such matters, the Judicial Council determined that resignation would be necessary if the organization involved itself directly or indirectly with health care concerns because continued participation would then constitute a voluntary professional association with cultists. As part of this broad interpretation of the chiropractic policy, the Judicial Council also ruled that a doctor would be guilty of unethical conduct even if he lectured to a group of chiropractors on medical subjects. Wilk defendant Joseph Sabatier (a member of the Committee on Quackery) once told a workshop of the Michigan State Medical Society that a medical doctor was unethical if he referred a patient to a chiropractor for *any* reason. The society subsequently resolved to inform its membership "that it is considered unethical by the AMA and, henceforth, by the MSMS [Michigan State Medical Society] for a doctor of medicine to refer a patient to a chiropractor for any reason."[45]

The AMA's net of influence extended even beyond constituent societies and individual doctors. The AMA was part owner of the Joint Commission on Accreditation of Hospitals (JCAH) along with the American College of Physicians, the American College of Surgeons, and the American Hospital Association, all codefendants in the Wilk case. Representatives from the latter three groups joined with the AMA to set requirements for JCAH accreditation. In 1971, the AMA suggested that JCAH incorporate a new interpretation of hospital accreditation into *Hospital Accreditation References*, its manual on standards. Adopted as standard 10, the measure required every hospital medical staff to form an ethics committee to enforce the ethical principles of the profession, defined in a footnote to mean the Principles and Medical Ethics of the AMA, which prohibited professional association with chiropractors. "Failure by the medical staff and the governing body [of a hospital] to take all reasonable steps to ensure adherence to these ethical principles," standard 10 warned, "shall constitute grounds for non-accreditation." In subsequent correspondence, JCAH made it clear to hospital administrators that, if they granted chiropractors privileges, accreditation would be withdrawn even if state legislation required hospitals to accept chiropractors as members of a medical staff.[46]

Consequently, hospitals refused to grant chiropractors access to hospital facilities and threatened physicians with loss of hospital privileges if they consulted with chiropractors. Wilk plaintiff Steven Lumsden was refused use of hospital x-ray and laboratory facilities at Helen Newberry Joy Hospital in Newberry, Michigan, because the medical staff felt denial to be "in the best interest of maintaining their status" with the JCAH. Plaintiff Patricia Arthur was denied benefit of x-ray equipment at a small Colorado hospital because the hospital attorney was fearful of losing accreditation, which would put the facility "in deep trouble." Subsequently, her patients had to travel sixty mountainous miles to the closest chiropractor with x-ray service. Plaintiff James Bryden of Sedalia, Missouri, routinely sent electrocardiogram tapes to Dr. Block, a local cardiologist, for interpretation. When rumors circulated that Block was associating with chiropractors, the Ethics Committee of the Bothwell Memorial Hospital summoned him for questioning. Block had read the electrocardiograms in his private office, yet the committee informed him that any commerce with a chiropractor was unethical according to JCAH standards and that continuing the practice would result in revocation of hospital privileges.[47]

On August 27, 1987, eleven years after the Wilk case first began, Federal Judge Susan Getzendanner rendered a decision after wading through some 1,265 exhibits, excerpts from 73 depositions, and 3,624 transcript pages. She found the AMA and its codefendants guilty of violating the Sherman Act through "a group boycott or conspiracy against chiropractors from 1966 to 1980, when principle 3 was finally eliminated." To determine whether or not the boycott involved an unreasonable restraint of trade, she applied the rule of reason. "The AMA's intent is clearly relevant to the rule of reason analysis," she held. "The boycott was intended to contain and eliminate the entire profession of chiropractic. Whether or not the elimination of chiropractic per se was consciously intended, that was the natural result of an intent to destroy a competitor." Because of the "substantial market power" of the AMA and its specific intent toward chiropractic, "a substantial adverse effect on competition is evident."

The AMA attempted to justify its conduct with a patient care defense. According to the guidelines previously determined by the Court of Appeals, a successful defense along these lines required the defendant to show that a genuine concern for the scientific method in patient care was the dominant motive, that it was objectively reasonable, and that such concern could not have been satisfied in a manner less restrictive of competition. Although Getzendanner determined that the defendant satisfied the first demand, she remained unimpressed with the AMA's sincerity. "I have some question," she observed, "about the genuineness of the AMA's concern for the scientific method based on the fact that when the AMA adopted changes in its chiropractic policies between 1977 and 1980, it apparently did so without deciding whether chiropractic was scientific. That shows disregard for scientific method in patient care." Based on extensive testimony regarding chiropractic effectiveness from witnesses on both sides (Getzendanner noted that "most of the defense witnesses, surprisingly, appeared to be testifying for the plaintiffs"), the court ruled that defendants' concern for the scientific method was not objectively reasonable for the duration of the boycott. On the final question of the patient care defense, she commented: "It would be a difficult task to persuade a court that a boycott and conspiracy designed to contain and eliminate a profession that was licensed in all fifty states at the time the Committee on Quackery disbanded was the only way to satisfy the AMA's concern for the use of scientific method in patient care." The AMA, continued Getzendanner, presented no evidence that a campaign of public education or any other less restrictive approach had been attempted and failed. Concern for the scientific method in patient care could have been satisfied in other, less suppressive ways. Based on these cumulative findings, she concluded that "the AMA has failed to carry its burden of persuasion on the patient care defense."[48]

For redress, Getzendanner agreed with the plaintiffs that an injunction was necessary.

> There are lingering effects of the conspiracy; the AMA has never acknowledged the lawlessness of its past conduct and in fact to this day maintains that it has always been in compliance with the antitrust laws; there has never been an affirmative statement by the AMA that it is ethical to associate with chiropractors; there has never been a public statement to AMA members of the admissions made in this court about the improved nature of chiropractic despite the fact that the AMA today claims that it made changes in its policy in recognition of the change and improvement in chiropractic; there has never been public retraction of articles such as "The Right and Duty of Hospitals to Deny Chiropractic Access to Hospitals"; a medical physician

has to very carefully read the current AMA Judicial Council Opinions to realize that there has been a change in the treatment of chiropractors and the court cannot assume that members of the AMA pore over these opinions; and finally, the systematic, long-term wrongdoing and the long-term intent to destroy a licensed profession suggests that an injunction is appropriate in this case.

Getzendanner ruled that among the defendants only the AMA, the American College of Surgeons, and the American College of Radiology were to be held liable for the boycott and conspiracy. She deemed the JCAH, the American College of Physicians, and the American Academy of Orthopaedic Surgeons to be innocent of overt conspiratorial intent even though they decidedly opposed chiropractic. The other original Wilk defendants had settled with the plaintiffs before this judgment and were no longer included in the suit.[49]

The court's Permanent Injunction Order restricted the AMA from interfering with the freedom of physicians and hospitals to make individual decisions regarding professional associations with chiropractors. The court directed the AMA to send a copy of the order by first class mail within thirty days of issuance to each member and employee, to publish the order in the *Journal of the American Medical Association,* and to modify the official AMA Judicial Council Opinions to reflect its current position given in court that physicians may associate professionally with chiropractors if deemed to be in the patient's best interest. In the final few days before the order was issued, the American College of Radiology and the American College of Physicians reached a settlement with the plaintiffs which ended further litigation. The AMA, however, filed an appeal, but in early 1990 the 7th U.S. Circuit Court of Appeals affirmed the finding of U.S. District Judge Susan Getzendanner.[50]

Although some chiropractors believed that the judgment against the AMA was too lenient, they all celebrated the decision as vindication and dubbed it the "Victory of the Century." "They don't have to love us, but they'll have to respect us and respect the law," Chester Wilk told the *Chiropractic Journal.* "There are laws in this land that say they can't do certain things, and they're not above the law. You can't just take the spots off the leopard and expect it to be tame. They'll still be dangerous, but at least they're not going to be so open because their lawyers are going to tell them 'shut up or you'll go to jail.' "[51]

The Wilk decision meant that chiropractors had organized medicine at bay and that the final barrier to legitimacy and cultural authority had eroded. The boost to chiropractic was immediate. A legislative bill in Michigan designed to relax restrictions on chiropractors easily passed in the House. The *American Medical News* reported that for Michigan legislators "the Wilk ruling has enhanced chiropractors' legitimacy and made physicians appear somewhat churlish."[52] Even before the Getzendanner decision, the Illinois State Medical Society, one of the original codefendants, had reached a settlement with the plaintiffs under which the society paid the plaintiffs $35,000 and permitted members to engage freely in interprofessional relations with chiropractors, including group practice in partnerships, HMOs, and other alternative health care delivery systems.[53]

Yet the symbolic chiropractic coup de grâce over medical authority came quietly when a chiropractor advertised for a physician in a small Detroit newspaper ("M.D. Wanted. Part time. Sixty-five dollars per hr. Busy Chiropractic Clinic") and easily filled the position. Chiropractors across the country routinely take dozens of applications for a single position and hire medical doctors on an hourly basis. This is the ultimate irony, much like chickens taking applications from destitute foxes to handle an overabundance of eggs in well-appointed and stylish coops. Chiropractor Philip Gray of Overland Park, Kansas, noted that, even without advertising, he is approached by physicians who ask to associate with him. "Medical doctors are looking for patients everywhere. If they had all the patients they could handle, you wouldn't see so much togetherness. . . . But the dollar," he concluded, "has the last say."[54]

Chapter Seven

Poetry with Science:
The Flourishing of Chiropractic

He's a different kind of doctor, but a doctor just the same,
Yet he doesn't have an M.D. as part of his printed name.
He spent years of work and study learning what makes people ill,
But he doesn't write prescriptions—and he doesn't give one pill.

What he does is fairly simple: he determines what is wrong
And then he adjusts our bodies, helping nature well along
To build up those weakened functions—to let nature take it's [sic]
   course.
Giving strength where it is needed through our nerve supply and
   source.

So the people come to see him and respond to gentle hands
As he guides them through their trouble, all because he understands
What their needs are. Now this doctor has a different degree;
He's your chiropractic doctor, with the title of D.C.

Anonymous

Street-level, his office is the one / between the Center for the Esoteric
   Arts / and the door announcing LAWYER. / The receptionist in
   white prefixes / every comment to him with a "Doctor" / as if she can
   award degrees.

Inside the conference room he asks / you things he has no right to
   know / and marks the answers on a scoresheet. / Examining, he
   smiles to see / the iron hand-grip barely register / your strain, he
   stretches you

until you call him uncle, / then puts you on a table tilting / like a
burial at sea. The largest man / who's ever stood above you says "Re-
lax" / and grabs you. Something cracks . . .

you're in the alleys of an ancient dream / where when you tried to
scream for help / no sound came out, you want to cry, / you want
to beat him up */ but you consented!*

The chiropractor can adjust you until / he's Atlas. This pain needs
movement— / off his table, on your feet and out the door / into the
dear humidity of Boston / carrying the body's grief on your back.

Carole Oles, "The Chiropractor"

Through the years, experiences with chiropractors have run the
gamut, from those who skip away from an adjustment in relief to those
who stumble back to the street bent in redoubled pain. But failures haunt
any brand of healers and, among the nonorthodox, chiropractors have
achieved unparalleled success. Current discussions of unorthodox therapies
often omit chiropractic among their subjects;[1] successful movements tend
to force redefinitions of orthodoxy. Because of its performance, chiropractic
has moved into position as the orthodox, nontraditional approach to
health—a type of orthodox unorthodoxy—and, emulating orthodoxy, has
assumed the full trappings of the medical establishment including the
"Dr." title, extended schooling, starched white coats, and magazine-stocked
offices complete with receptionists and insurance adjusters.

Chiropractic now occupies a unique, middle ground between regular
medicine and the harmonial-style therapies of the holistic health movement
that have blossomed in the past quarter century. The struggle of chiropractic has been part of the larger, continuing struggle over the nature of
science and the relationship between *spiritus* and *materia,* a battle that the
Matter-directed rationality of the mechanical tradition has dominated since
the end of the seventeenth century. The harmonial impulse, imbued with
the intuition that Matter and Spirit were intimately bound, reemerged in
Mesmerism and the magnetic healing movements of the nineteenth century, reminding the scientific community, as did William James, that the
purposes of science "are not the only purposes, and that the order of
uniform causation which she has use for, and is therefore right in postulat-
ing, may be enveloped in a wider order, on which she has no claim at all."[2]
Original chiropractic stood in the vanguard of a popular harmonialism
reemerging in late nineteenth-century America, a movement dissatisfied
with the limits of a mechanical approach to the world. Chiropractic joined
the realms of Spirit (in the Palmers' notions of Universal, Innate, and
Educated Intelligence) with the realms of Matter (in a practical technique

for relieving pain). Chiropractic promised to salve both the religious longings and the physical ailments of disgruntled Americans.

As with any movement, chiropractic changed with development. A number of early chiropractors became unsettled with the Palmer ideology and sought to remake chiropractic in the image of modern science by focusing on Matter. These mechanics within the movement began to dominate and attempted to attach a modern, scientific rationale to their manipulations. Throughout, the harmonists retained a strong and vocal presence in the tradition of the Palmers and forged a natural bond with the holistic health reformers of the past few decades. For example, chiropractor Mark Grinims joined with Walter Fischman, a doctor of Chinese medicine, to develop a test of arm-strength known as "the muscle response test," which is related to Chinese acupuncture points and "lines of energy" that reputedly tap the body's own curative powers. The therapist determines the need for specific vitamins and minerals by touching particular parts of the body and testing the strength of the opposite arm. Points of correspondence between body and vitamin have been determined by "intuitive knowledge." The right eyelid, for example, is the spot for vitamin A; if the subject's left arm is weak when the reader touches the eyelid, the body is crying out for vitamin A. To determine proper dosage, the patient adds small increments of the indicated vitamin or mineral to his mouth or hand. The arm muscle becomes strong when the correct amount is held; an excessive dose will cause the muscle to again weaken.[3] Chiropractor Carl Ferreri developed a variation of the muscle strength test called neural organization technique (NOT), which employs skull as well as spinal adjustments. Ferreri claims success in treating children with dyslexia, Down's syndrome, cerebral palsy, scoliosis, bedwetting and bowel problems, colorblindness, and nightmares while freeing them from fear and stimulating emotional growth and physical agility. In a recent experiment sponsored by the Del Norte County (Cal.) Unified School District, NOT chiropractors treated dozens of children and set off a storm of controversy between parents who claimed that NOT had seriously harmed their children and those who rejoiced at dramatic improvement.[4]

Escondido chiropractor Bernard Jensen is currently the most widely quoted American practitioner of iridology (a belief that the eye's iris is the key to diagnosing bodily ills, changing in color and texture when a problem develops in any organ system) and has published two textbooks heavily laced with New Age ideology. California chiropractor John F. Thie has developed "Touch for Health," a blend of Palmer chiropractic and acupressure that touts the connection of Innate with Universal Intelligence.[5]

Although such approaches are anathema to mechanics within the profession, the continuing schism with harmonists, while painful and acrimonious, means that chiropractic can appeal both to the modern scientific

community because of recent studies indicating the value of spinal manipulation *and* to the holistic health and "New Age" sensibilities because of
its harmonial heritage and its all-natural "no drug, no bug, no surgery"
orientation. Chiropractors can comfortably don either the cloaks of Mesmer or the labcoats of the clinician.

Chiropractic also grew up alongside high technology. John Naisbitt
argued that the escalation of high technology within a society creates a
compensatory need for "high touch," a counterbalancing human response,
"soft edges" that counteract the "hard edges of technology."[6] Chiropractic
is high touch in a very literal as well as emotional sense. The core of
chiropractic work is touching and listening, validating the often ambiguous
pain associated with back ailments. As high technology entered the medical
marketplace, physicians focused increasingly on parts rather than patients,
on Matter rather than Spirit and emotion. At the same time that specialization engendered by high technology served to make doctors' cures more
certain, it also served to undermine the emotional and psychological dependency of the patient on the physician. In a recent round table discussion
among physicians and consultants reported in *Medical Economics,* internist
Walter O'Donnell noted "the absolute, primeval need people have to turn
to some strong person who they believe can help them. The physician
who relies on fancy technology or on physician extenders [such as nurse
practitioners] isn't giving that to his patients." Agreeing with O'Donnell,
general surgeon Leonard Deitz responded: "We have increasing pressure
for depersonalized medicine and I think doctors must resist. It's an attitude
that first takes root in medical school. The residents I teach, for instance,
don't have 'patients.' They have 'cases.' "[7] High-tech instruments and procedures have moved physicians away from high-touch practice, placing a
barrier between doctor and patient. Physicians tend to concentrate on
disease, the tangible damage suffered by a body, rather than *illness,* the
broader, subjective experience of sickness. Chiropractors, in contrast, focus
on illness and treat by touching, talking, listening, accepting, supporting,
and creating hope[8]—all of the high-touch activities that physicians have
frequently neglected in the celebration of high technology.

Chiropractic survived and flourished ultimately because it "worked"
for large numbers of people; although necessary, this alone was insufficient
to sustain it, since other alternative therapies, such as Thomsonianism,
hydropathy, homeopathy, and osteopathy, have also "worked" at some
level for many.[9] Alternative health movements, like third parties in American politics, tend to rise when the establishment fails to address widespread
concerns brewing within the public. Americans in the early nineteenth
century were distressed by the "heroic" practices of orthodox medicine,
the excessive bleedings and blisterings, purgings and pukings that seemed
to create more troubles than solutions. Thomsonianism, hydropathy, and

homeopathy became antidotes to the heroic measures, offering more therapeutically conservative remedies to a public suspicious of orthodoxy. Even
though doctors delighted in ridiculing these alternatives, the medical marketplace forced them to reappraise their own armamentarium and eventually to abandon the harshest of the heroic practices. A convergence began,
with the orthodox edging toward the competition while the alternatives
deserted their own extremes and moved toward the regulars. Orthodox
medical practice both expanded and contracted, absorbing within its own
arsenal the best offered by the other healers and expelling the worst. The
move of regular doctors toward therapeutic nihilism in the middle third of
the century meant that Nature, which had underwritten the cures of the
alternative healers, was now also in the camp of the orthodox. Much like
a major political party co-opting the particular issues raised by a third party,
orthodox medicine absorbed and co-opted the alternative healers whose
distinctiveness and *raison d'être* began to vanish.

Osteopathy and chiropractic, arising near the end of the century,
presented a somewhat different challenge for the regulars. These two movements offered a distinctive therapy—manual manipulation—rejected by
American orthodoxy as unworthy of consideration. Manipulation, unlike
the milder drugs, curative waters, and dietary reforms touted by earlier
alternative healers, was foreign to regular doctors and required considerable
skill to master. Because the monistic claims of the manipulators struck
physicians as outlandish and even embarrassing, they resorted to ridicule
and had no desire to incorporate manipulative skills within orthodox practice, especially at a time when science through the microscope was revealing
the specific causes of particular diseases and offering designer drugs to
overpower the offending microorganisms. The passivity of trusting Nature
was giving way to a new medical activism among the regulars. Manipulators
seemed excessively crude and simplistic by comparison to the emerging
complexity of medical understanding. Osteopaths eventually responded to
derision by becoming more like medical doctors, abandoning manipulation
as an exclusive focus. Andrew Taylor Still, the originator of osteopathy,
had trained as a medical doctor; because of this background, a retreat to
orthodoxy was a logical step for osteopathy in the face of excessive hostility
and abuse from the regulars. Osteopaths survived by becoming virtually
indistinguishable from doctors of medicine on terms proffered by the
medical profession.

Chiropractic, brainchild of D.D. and B.J. Palmer, had no such medical heritage to tap. Physicians, who viewed chiropractic as a comical, cheap
knock-off of osteopathy, refused to offer fellowship on any terms. When
ridicule rained from the doctors, chiropractors faced only two choices—
disband the movement or become even more zealous. Convinced that they
were armed with the Truth of Health, chiropractic advocates refused to

capitulate to medical taunting and chose the latter course, developing a staunch, belligerent posture that served to carry the movement through difficult times. Despite intramural conflict and bickering centered largely around B.J. Palmer, chiropractic developed a unity spurred by incessant medical opposition, a psychological brotherhood of the dumped-upon. D.D. Palmer himself clearly understood the phenomenon. From his Scott County, Iowa, jail cell in 1906, he developed a maxim to instill disheartened followers with optimism: "Persecution or prosecution creates sympathy, sympathy generates investigators, investigation produces followers, who become more zealous and persistent in spreading their peculiar doctrines." Intuitively, Palmer sensed that many Americans possessed the French *esprit frondeur*—a tendency to disagree with the establishment—and delighted in cheering for the Davids of the world.[10] Chiropractic survived, in large part, *because* of medical hostility and legal harassment.

A convergence of other factors also served to buttress chiropractic. In the first two decades of the twentieth century, Progressive reformers of all stripes demanded efficiency above all else. James Whorton noted that, "despite the significant differences in their individual programs of physical salvation, Progressive health reformers spoke a *lingua franca* in which the crucial adjectives were natural, harmonious, evolutionary, successful, and efficient."[11] Although Progressive reformers such as Abraham Flexner and Morris Fishbein denounced chiropractic as tomfoolery, it nevertheless scored well by the measures of efficiency they cherished. What could be more compatible with the demands of efficiency than an ideology that stressed the harmony of Spirit and Matter and offered success with a natural, drugless technique that cured with a swift, low-cost adjustment? Unwittingly, Progressive rhetoric, along with a growing public suspicion of drugs also fueled by Progressives, served to sustain chiropractic.[12]

Chiropractic also benefited from dwindling numbers of physicians in the first third of the century and the concurrent medical exodus from rural to urban areas, a reapportionment of physicians dictated by the population requirements of increasing specialization. In many rural areas, chiropractors became primary care-givers with little competition from the orthodox. In urban areas, chiropractors also survived because they were glad to treat patients with chronic, often ambiguous pain that medical doctors came to view as an unprofitable drain on their time and resources. Medical specialism meant clear-cut solutions for particular, well-defined ailments. Nagging backaches, usually immune to diagnosis through sophisticated technology, remained outside the realm of medical mastery.

Chiropractic, like any alternative healing movement, could survive as long as it offered a distinctive therapy alien to the orthodox that created dependency among patients for its services. The *widespread* dependency that chiropractic achieved meant that chiropractic success, in a limited sense, came before chiropractors had garnered a significant measure of legitimacy. But therapeutic success alone cannot generate the necessary cultural authority for a modern movement to flourish. Without legitimacy achieved according to the rules of modern science, chiropractic, despite its record of success, would have remained only a marginal discipline consigned to the medical underworld inhabited by other heterodox healers. Truly to flourish rather than merely to survive, a twentieth-century health movement must create authority officially recognized by state and federal governments and by health insurance companies. Accruing this cultural authority requires more than a demonstration of patient dependency—it demands legitimacy measured by the standards and rationale of modern science. Successful and controlled clinical testing explained by sensible theory is the modern pathway to legitimacy Within the last two decades, reinforced by kudos from the popular press, chiropractic has been able to withstand the scrutiny required to achieve legitimacy. A chiropractic substructure of success was in place—by 1974, licensing laws secured in all fifty states and an educational establishment (rid of inferior proprietary schools) that boasted its own federally sanctioned accrediting agency. With chiropractic care now covered under state and federal workmen's compensation plans, Medicare and Medicaid, and most commercial health carriers, chiropractors have achieved the Holy Grail of health professionals, third-party reimbursement. Along with medical doctors, chiropractors have themselves become gatekeepers to health.

This chiropractic accomplishment, of course, was far from inevitable. Any description of a successful movement tends to lend a sense of inevitability and false clarity to the complex, confusing fits and starts that participants actually experienced. Stated simply (perhaps too simply), enough chiropractors eventually learned how to play the modern game of legitimacy, based ultimately on their therapeutic success, that official recognition came. An erstwhile medical pariah, chiropractic has flourished in modern America and continues to grow rapidly.[13]

The library at Logan College of Chiropractic in Chesterfield, Missouri, is housed in what was formerly the Chapel of the Maryknoll Seminary. In the rear next to study tables, five full skeletons and two spines dangle in front of spired windows still resplendent in colorful, intricate patterns of stained glass. The spines and stained glass seem at first incongruous, but chiropractic success ultimately hinged on just such a combination—stained glass with spinal manipulation, Spirit with Matter, Poetry with Science. "Nothing is more dangerous than science without poetry, technical progress without emotional content," H. St. Chamberlain has argued. "The proof lies in the hypertrophied intellectuality and rationality of our own age, and the simultaneous degeneration of sentiment to the sub-human level."[14] Although falling far short of D.D. Palmer's original millennial vision, chiropractic has retained a strong subculture of harmonialism while becoming an institutionalized part of America's health care system, a unique accomplishment among nineteenth-century alternative movements.

Postscript

Prospects for the Future of Chiropractic

ACA [American Chiropractic Association] reaffirms its position that chiropractic must be preserved as a separate and distinct branch of the healing arts.

ACA Intraprofessional Policy

Although chiropractic has arrived as an institutionalized part of America's health care system, arrival does not automatically confer permanent success nor continued cultural authority. Medical movements as well as individuals operate in a dynamic world of constant flux. For semantic clarity we tend to reify terms that help bring some order to this flow. The terms *cultural authority* and *legitimacy* are not single nor static things in themselves that a person or group either possesses or not. They are merely *descriptive* terms of relative status within a dynamic scene. There are numerous ill-defined levels and multiple layers of legitimacy and cultural authority; chiropractic has managed to scale some but not others. Legally, chiropractors have the full measure of authority to practice, yet an aura of quackery still lingers, haunting from the past.[1] Although difficult to differentiate precisely, the legitimacy and cultural authority attached to chiropractors are clearly different from those attached to medical doctors.

Chiropractors have also attained a type of professional status but one that is also different from that of their medical counterparts. Professionalism itself is not simply a bar, set at a static and predetermined height, that aspiring professionals must jump. As medical historian Martin Pernick aptly noted, the *content* of professionalism can change dramatically through time because of technological innovations or because of shifts in social values. Mundane, mainstream professional practices from two hundred years ago that inflicted wincing pain would be branded today as outrageously barbaric. Professionalism, Pernick argued, "is a changing ideology, one that demands very different attitudes and behavior from practitioners at different times."[2] The nineteenth-century medical profession, which focused on systems, was different from but not *inherently* less professional than its twentieth-century counterpart, which has focused on specialization. The ground undergirding "the professional" has shifted. Chiropractic, emerging at the turn of the century, was oriented toward systems at a time when medical professionalism demanded specialization. But even this simplifies. Chiropractic experienced a double dynamic—not only were notions of professionalism changing but also chiropractic itself was changing and stretching, sometimes reacting against the shifts and sometimes embracing them in an attempt to gain status according to newer definitions of professionalism. The current result is a somewhat curious mix. Chiropractors are professional spine specialists still geared toward holistic, systemic logic. Chiropractors *are* professionals, of a sort, and *have* legitimacy and cultural authority, of a sort. Chiropractors *have* achieved success, of a sort.

Given the successes of chiropractic to date, what are the prospects for the future? Where is chiropractic likely to head? Ten years ago, sociologist Walter Wardwell offered five different possible outcomes for chiropractic.

1. Complete fusion with medicine, following the path taken by homeopathy and osteopathy.
2. Practice under medical supervision, analogous to the role of physical therapists.
3. Disappearance of chiropractic and chiropractors.
4. Continuation of present distinctions, separate from medicine but marginal or even parallel to it.
5. Development as a limited medical profession, independent of medical supervision but limited in scope. Dentists could serve as a prestigious role model.

Of these possibilities, Wardwell believed that outcomes 1, 2, and 3 are highly unlikely and that outcome 4 or 5 is a real possibility, to be determined largely by what chiropractors themselves desire. As he noted correctly, however, chiropractors alone cannot determine their future (in the same way, it should be added, that they have not been the sole determinants of their past).[3]

The future has a way of chastening soothsayers. Nevertheless, my own assessment is that chiropractic will remain separate and decidedly distinct from orthodox medicine, neither marginal nor parallel. Chiropractic is already far beyond marginal by any reasonable measure, yet it seems unlikely (especially in the short term) that chiropractic will be able completely to shed the old stigma of chiro*quactic* that would allow it to emerge as truly parallel, invested with the cultural authority, legitimacy, and professional status enjoyed by medical doctors.

Fusion with orthodox medicine would provide one avenue to acquiring the status chiropractors lack. Yet chiropractic is unlikely to fuse with orthodox medicine as a means of gaining status partly because of the continuing rift in chiropractic ranks between what I have called harmonists and mechanics. If anything, the quasi-medical posturing of the mechanics is intensifying the desire of harmonists to fight vehemently against any chiropractic trend they view as diluting the original tenets and practices of the Palmers. The chiropractic journals are full of neofundamentalist appeals for "Revival in Chiropractic" which embrace the old-time views. For example, an ad for the "Living Principles Program" noted an alarming trend in chiropractic "toward physical medicine, physiotherapy, treatment and diagnosis of disease and the actual step toward teaching the chiropractor Materia Medica and surgery. . . . We, in LIVING PRINCIPLES are dedicated and devoted to the survival of chiropractic and . . . will be directing all our energies to keeping it VITALLY ALIVE!! . . . Together our eventual ultimate goal is to bring *unadulterated chiropractic to the world*" (emphasis in original).[4] Several neofundamentalist chiropractic colleges, such as Sherman College of Straight Chiropractic in Spartanburg, South Carolina, are dedicated *explicitly* to maintaining chiropractic as a distinct and separate discipline. This strong harmonial resurrection within chiropractic orients these chiropractors to the Palmer legacy and focuses on differences rather than similarities with orthodox medicine.

Although it is theoretically possible that the mechanics could break away from the harmonists and thoroughly embrace the medical profession, this is also highly unlikely. Despite the inflated rhetoric of the neofundamentalists, harmonists and mechanics have a much greater interest in remaining loosely together. At the same time, the very real divisions within chiropractic ranks will keep them from presenting a united front that might make a rapprochement with chiropractic appealing to medical doctors. With the Wilk decision and chiropractic inroads into the institutional structure of American health care, chiropractors are finally emerging from the ghetto mentality engendered by years of medical hostility and harassment. As George P. McAndrews, principal attorney for Wilk, argued recently, "It is especially important now for chiropractors to stay informed as chiropractic takes the offensive against the medical profession, which suddenly finds itself on the run."[5] Chiropractors are unlikely to let this advantage wither. Their distinctive skill, spinal manipulation, is still often disparaged by physicians and will continue to work toward keeping chiropractors separate and distinct from the medical profession. Many chiropractors continue to believe that M.D. is an abbreviation for **M**ajor **D**eity syndrome. Any animosity between chiropractors is trifling compared with the animosity between chiropractic and medicine.

Nevertheless, one possible avenue that could create chiropractic subservience to orthodox medicine would be the wholesale entry of chiropractors into hospitals, a former barrier eradicated by the Wilk case. Chiropractic groups hold "Chiropractic and Hospital Privileges" seminars designed both for chiropractors and hospital administrators. Entry into hospitals puts chiropractors on medical turf, subordinate to medical protocol within the hospital. For this reason, many chiropractors remain leery of hospital privileges. As Richard H. Tyler explained,

> There are some chiropractors who feel that to be an "RD" (real doctor) you have to be in a hospital at all costs. . . . It is . . . difficult for me to lower myself into a secondary position so that I may be "allowed" to admit a patient to a hospital. We are expected to hold on to big brother's hand and hope they'll let us in for half price. If you make it then you'd better be a good boy. . . .
>
> Yes—there is a need for in-patient hospital care—but is it worth your soul? You bet I'd be the first in line to get in—when the admitting doctor is Marcus Welby, D.C.
>
> Remember, the majority of those running the medical hospitals hate our guts. Only because they need the money our patients might bring in will they even deign to consider an association of any kind. So let's get off our knees and keep in mind that it's better to have broken knuckles from fighting for what you believe in than blood on your knees from begging.[6]

Chiropractors are a proud lot, unlikely to beg hospitals for anything. Chiropractors will be entering hospitals in ever-increasing numbers, but primarily on their own terms.[7] Subordinance within the hospital structure is improbable.

In sum, the most plausible outcome for chiropractic is medical *style* combined with chiropractic *substance*, best symbolized by the term *chiropractic physician* many chiropractors have adopted. By outliving and outperforming all of its nineteenth-century nonorthodox brethren, chiropractic represents a unique accomplishment. Neither marginal nor parallel to orthodox medicine, chiropractic will continue to occupy a unique niche.

Appendix A

Chiropractic Licensing Laws

Chronological Grouping of Chiropractic Licensing Statutes	Year Initial Law Passed	Composition of Chiropractic Licensing Board and Number of Board Members*
Before 1920		
Kansas	1913	A3 & B2[a]
North Dakota	1913	A5
Arkansas	1915	A3
Oregon	1915	A3
Nebraska	1915	X
Colorado	1915[b]	A5
Ohio	1915	B7[c]
North Carolina	1917	A3
Connecticut	1917	A3
Montana	1918	A3
Vermont	1919	A3
Minnesota	1919	A5
Idaho	1919	A3
Washington	1919	A3
1920–1929		
New Jersey	1920[d]	A1 & B10
Kentucky	1920	A3
Maryland	1920	A3
Arizona	1921	A3
New Mexico	1921	A3
Oklahoma	1921	A3
Iowa	1921	A3
South Dakota	1921	A
New Hampshire	1921	A3

Georgia	1921	A5
California	1922	A5
Virginia	1922	AB
Nevada	1923	A5
Illinois	1923	B5
Maine	1923	A5
Florida	1923	A3
Tennessee	1923	A3
Utah	1923	A
Wyoming	1924	A3
Hawaii	1925	X
Wisconsin	1925	X
West Virginia	1925	A2, B8, C1
Missouri	1927	A5
Rhode Island	1927	A2 & B1
Indiana	1927	A1 & B[e]
District of Columbia	1929	X
1930–1939		
South Carolina	1932	A4
Michigan	1933	A3
Delaware	1937	A3
Alaska	1938	X
After 1939		
Texas	1949	A9
Pennsylvania	1951	A5 & C1
Alabama	1960	A
New York	1963	A4 & B3[f]
Massachusetts	1966	A3 & B2
Mississippi	1973	X
Louisiana	1974	X

SOURCES: Phylis Lan Lin, "The Chiropractor, Chiropractic, and Process: A Study of the Sociology of an Occupation" (Ph.D. diss., University of Missouri-Columbia, 1972), 322–23; Andrew K. Berger, "A Chronology of Chiropractic Licensing in the United States and the District of Columbia," *Research Forum: A Journal of Chiropractic Research* 3 (Spring 1987): 78–83; Chittenden Turner, *The Rise of Chiropractic* (Los Angeles: Powell Publishing Co., 1931), 95–98, 338, 350, 364–65; Martha M. Metz, *Fifty Years of Chiropractic Recognized in Kansas* (Abilene, Kans.: Shadinger-Wilson, 1965), 94; Walter I. Wardwell, "The Cutting Edge of Chiropractic Recognition: Prosecution and Legislation in Massachusetts," *Chiropractic History* 2 (1982): 64; James G. Burrow, *Organized Medicine in the Progressive Era: The Move toward Monopoly* (Baltimore: Johns Hopkins University Press, 1977), 70.

Key: A, chiropractors; B, members of other occupations specified by law; C, ex-officio members; X, composition unknown.

[a] A minister and a school teacher were the specified nonchiropractic members.

[b] Licensed under the state medical board from 1915 through 1933.

[c] Schools of practice at variance with the regulars were given representation in proportion to their numerical strength in the state, but no school could have a majority.

[d] Repealed the 1920 act sometime before 1924 and repassed it in 1953.

[e] The lone chiropractor sat with the medical board.

[f] The nonchiropractic members were a medical doctor, a New York University scientist, and an osteopath.

Appendix B

Chiropractic Articles in the Popular Periodical Press

Arriving at a comprehensive definition of the popular periodical press is a difficult and elusive task. Here the term refers to those publications that achieved widespread circulation and were intended for a general, educated audience. As a practical matter, the *Readers' Guide to Periodical Literature,* the *Popular Periodicals Index,* and the online *Infotrac—Magazine Index* served as the principal means for locating articles concerning chiropractic. I located a few through textual clues in indexed articles and a few by serendipity. Two basic questions guided the analysis: What has been the reputation or "image" of chiropractic in the periodical press? What might this image have to do with the survival of chiropractic? In addition, the second question implies a third: What influence can be attributed to the popular periodical press?

I used a five-tier classification of the articles as the means for understanding the reputation of chiropractic in the popular press. I classified the "tone" of each article as either extremely negative ($--$), negative ($-$), neutral (0), positive ($+$), or extremely positive ($++$) (see the table). I decided to use a five-tier scheme rather than a simpler three-tier approach (of negative, neutral, positive) because five categories could capture the tone of the articles more accurately. I used the double-negative designation when the article acknowledged no redeeming virtue in chiropractice. Articles that were basically skeptical but admitted the possibility that chiropractic might be of some limited benefit to a few received the single negative. Neutral pieces were those that discussed the merits and deficiencies of chiropractic in a reasoned manner without endorsement or condemnation. I used the single positive when the article endorsed chiropractic without viewing it as a medical panacea. Articles receiving the double positive did not necessarily see chiropractic as a cure-all (although some did), but endorsed it wholeheartedly as a legitimate healing art and deserving of acceptance and recognition. As a check on my assessments, I had two readers independently rate some of the articles and then matched the ratings with my own. One read forty-seven articles and agreed completely with my evaluation on forty-one (an 87 percent agreement rate), and the second read ten articles with eight total agreements (80 percent). The few disagreements that did occur were minimal. In only one case was a disagreement two categories apart; the other disagreements were only one category apart.

Some writers immediately negated any suspense by using titles such as "Chiroquactic" (*Hygeia*, December 1948), "Visit to a Bizarre World— Chiropractic Alma Maters" (*Today's Health*, July 1968), or the more bland but straightforward entries in the February 1950 *American Mercury*, "The Case against Chiropractic," and "The Case for Chiropractic." Section headings and subtitles occasionally tipped the reader to the tone of the article. "Spinal Discord," in the August 1974 issue of *Money*, came in a section labeled "The Angry Consumer." Subtitles such as "Nine Million Patients Can't All Be Wrong" in the December 1978 issue of *Family Health* and "The Long-Misunderstood Profession Is Making a Comeback" in the April 1984 *Esquire* indicated that positive assessments followed. Cartoons, photographs, and diagrams also accompanied some articles and frequently served to reinforce the tenor of the argument. Cartoons became vehicles for expressing negative opinions of chiropractic, whereas photographs and diagrams tended to carry complimentary messages. In short, the classification process was relatively easy because of a lack of subtlety among the writers.

CHIROPRACTIC ARTICLES IN THE POPULAR PERIODICAL PRESS IN CHRONOLOGICAL SEQUENCE

Magazine	Date of Publication	Article Title	Author	Tone of Article	Circulation[a]	Percentage of U.S. Population Represented by Circulation[b]
Harper's Weekly	Mar. 27, 1915	"Drug Doctors' and the 'Medical Trust'"	George Creel	− −	39,956	0.04
Harper's Weekly	Apr. 3, 1915	"Making Doctors While You Wait"	George Creel	− −	39,956	0.04
Harper's Weekly	Apr. 10, 1915	"Mail Order Miracle Men"	George Creel	− −	39,956	0.04
Harper's Weekly	Apr. 24, 1915	"Easy Money Doctors"	George Creel	− −	39,956	0.04
Harper's Weekly	Sept. 18, 1915	"Chiropractic Backbone"	Lyndon E. Lee, D.C.	+ +	39,956	0.04
Overland Monthly	Apr. 1920	"Where Doctors Differ"	Frederick L. Douglas	−	64,863	0.06
Scientific American	May 1922	"Doctors and Near-Doctors"	Not given	− −	c. 90,000	0.08
Atlantic Monthly	July 1922	"Osteopathy, Chiropractic, and the Profession of Medicine"	Channing Froth-ingham	−	c. 107,000	0.1
Scientific American	Aug. 1923	"The Possibilities of Sub-luxations"	Ray G. Hulburt, D.O.	−	c. 90,000	0.08
American Mercury	May 1925	"Chiropractic"	Morris Fishbein, [M.D.]	− −	69,278	0.06
American Mercury	Jan. 1931	"The Chiropractor"	Albert Lindsay O'Neale, Jr.	− −	62,074	0.05
Time	Mar. 18, 1940	"Cosmic Chiropractor"	Not given	−	759,520	0.6
Hygeia (reprinted in abridged form, June 1946 Reader's Digest)	Apr. 1946	"Can Chiropractic Cure?"	Albert Q. Maisel	− −	151,508	0.1

CHIROPRACTIC ARTICLES (Continued)

Magazine	Date of Publication	Article Title	Author	Tone of Article	Circulation[a]	Percentage of U.S. Population Represented by Circulation[b]
Ebony	Dec. 1946	"School for Chiropractors"	Not given	+	324,930 [for 1947; not listed for 1946]	0.2
Reader's Digest	Feb. 1947	"Chiropractic Presents Its Case"	C. W. Weiant, D.C.	+ +	3,080,000	2.1
Time	Mar. 17, 1947	"It's All in the Spine"	Not given	– –	1,586,015	1.1
Hygeia	Dec. 1948	"Chiroquactic"	Morris Fishbein, [M.D.]	– –	195,387	0.1
American Mercury	Feb. 1950	"The Case against Chiropractic"	Joseph D. Wassersug, M.D.	– –	40,804	0.03
American Mercury	Feb. 1950	"The Case for Chiropractic"	Sherman Levin	+ +	40,804	0.03
Newsweek	Feb. 6, 1950	"Chiropractic. Pro and Con"		–	836,305	0.6
American Mercury	Apr. 1950	"Chiropractic—For and Against" (three letters to the editor)	1. L.W. Zarrell, D.C., Ph.C. 2. Sherman Levin 3. Joseph D. Wassersug, M.D.	+ + + + – –	40,804	0.03
Cosmopolitan	Dec. 1953	"Chiropractic—Science or Quackery?"	James Phelan	0	1,697,900	1.1
Man's Magazine	Apr. 1955	"The Truth about Chiropractors"	Thorp McClusky	+ +	197,528 [for 1956]	0.1
Good Housekeeping	June 1958	"Osteopaths and Chiropractors Are Not the Same"	Not given	0	4,367,766	2.5
McCalls	Oct. 1959	"The Case for the Chiropractors"	Samuel Grafton	+ +	5,491,572	3.1
Newsweek	Apr. 8, 1963	"Foot in the Door"	Not given	–	1,600,948	0.8

Magazine	Date	Title	Author		Circulation	
Life	Apr. 9, 1965	"If Your Back Is Out, You're 'In'"	Marshall Smith	0	7,327,185	3.8
Today's Health	May 1965	"Chiropractic: Science or Swindle?"	Ralph Lee Smith	− −	702,419	0.4
Science	Mar. 11, 1966	Letter to the Editor	C.W. Weiant, D.C.	+ +	121,490	0.06
Science	June 3, 1966	"Chiropractic Education" (two letters to the editor)	1. Henry Fineberg, M.D. 2. J. Sabatier	− −	121,490	0.06
Good Housekeeping	May 1967	"The Medical Dispute about Treatment by Chiropractors"	Not given	−	5,500,000[c]	2.8
Today's Health	June 1968	"Golden Touch for Chiropractors"	Ralph Lee Smith	− −	710,000[c]	0.4
Today's Health	July 1968	"Visit to a Bizarre World—Chiropractic Alma Maters"	Ralph Lee Smith	− −	710,000[c]	0.4
Today's Health	Apr. 1969	"HEW Rejects Chiropractic"	Not given	− −	710,000[c]	0.4
Today's Health	Jan. 1970	"Chiropractic: Issues and Answers"	Ralph Lee Smith and Joseph A. Sabatier, M.D.	− −	710,000[d]	0.3
Mechanix Illustrated	Apr. 1971	"What Can a Chiropractor Do for You"	Lester David	0	1,500,000[d]	0.7
Reader's Digest	July 1971	"Should Chiropractors Be Paid with Your Tax Dollars?"	Albert Q. Maisel	− −	17,829,000[d]	8.6
Ladies Home Journal	Nov. 1972	"Do Chiropractors Really Help You?"	Jack H. Pollack	+ +	7,000,000[d]	3.4
Money	Aug. 1974	"Spinal Discord"	Robert M. Randall	− −	600,000[e]	0.3
Science	Sept. 1974	"Chiropractic: Healing or Hokum? HEW is Looking for Answers"	Constance Holden	0	149,557[e]	0.07
Prevention	Apr. 1975	"Chiropractic vs. M.D.'s: Which Is Better for Back Pain?"	Not given	+ +	1,600,000[e]	0.7

CHIROPRACTIC ARTICLES (Continued)

Magazine	Date of Publication	Article Title	Author	Tone of Article	Circulation[a]	Percentage of U.S. Population Represented by Circulation[b]
Consumer Reports	Sept. 1975	"Chiropractors: Healers or Quacks? Part I: The 80 Year War with Science"	[Joseph Botta]	−	2,300,000[a]	1.1
Consumer Reports	Oct. 1975	"Part II: How Chiropractic Can Help—or Harm"	Not given	−	2,300,000[a]	1.1
Psychology Today	Feb. 1976	"The Chiropractic Controversy"	Jack Horn	+	1,000,000[e]	0.5
Family Health	Dec. 1978	"Chiropractic Comes of Age"	Joseph B. Treaster	+	1,000,000[e]	0.5
Prevention	Mar. 1979	"Dr. Hatfield-McCoy"	John Yates	+ +	1,600,000[e]	0.7
Good Housekeeping		"Chiropractors: What They Can and Can't Do for You"				2.3
Sports Illustrated	Apr. 1979	"Good Hands Man: Sports Chiropractor"	E.R. Mark	+	c. 5,000,000[f]	0.9
Dance Magazine	July 16, 1979	"What the Chiropractor Can Do for the Dancer"	Herman Weiskopf	+ +	c. 2,000,000[f]	0.03
Prevention	Jan. 1980	"A Case of Chronic Headache"	Margaret Pierpont	+ +	60,000[f]	0.9
	Feb. 1980		Jonathan V. Wright, M.D.	+ +	c. 2,000,000[f]	
Runner's World	Sept. 1980	"Runner's World Exclusive: The Gadfly of the AMA, Dr. Leroy Perry [D.C.] Mixes Medicine and Motivational Magic"	Not given	+ +	325,000[f]	0.14
FDA Consumer	Mar. 1981	"Public Disservice Announcement"	Not given	− −	30,000[a] includes paid and nonpaid	0.01

Magazine	Date	Article	Author		Circulation	
Scientific News	May 16, 1981	"Spine Manipulation for Low Back Pain"	Not given	+	Not listed	0.9
Glamour	June 1981	"Chiropractors: Can They Really Help You?"	Richard Trubo	+	2,003,882[a]	1.2
Cosmopolitan	Feb. 1982	"Chiropractic and You: (It Couldn't Hurt to Find Out!)"	Grant Pick	+	2,747,042[f]	
Health	Mar. 1982	"Chiropractic's New Twist"	Dalma Heyn	++	846,615[a]	0.4
Prevention	Mar. 1984	"Hands-On Health: An Illustrated Guide to the Manipulative Arts"	Kerry Pechter	++	2,821,501[g]	1.2
Mother Earth News	Mar./Apr. 1984	"Spontaneous Release by Positioning"	Andrew Saul	++	984,599[a]	0.4
Esquire	Apr. 1984	"The Chiropractor: The Long Misunderstood Profession is Making a Comeback"	Barbara Kelves	++	730,615[a]	0.3
Dance Magazine	Sept. 1984	"Body Health: What Cracks While Cracking"	Lawrence F. DeMann, D.C.	++	52,812[a] includes paid and nonpaid	0.02
Bicycling	Nov./Dec. 1984	"Spinal Manipulation: A New Twist"	Maria Mihalik	+	253,373[g]	0.11
McCalls	Dec. 1984	"Straight Talk about Chiropractors"	Madeline Chinnici et al.	+	c. 6,500,000[f]	2.7
Reader's Digest	Jan. 1985	"Good News about Bad Backs"	Claire Safran	+	18,000,000[g]	7.5
Newsweek	Aug. 12, 1985	"A New Medical Marriage"	Eileen Keerdoja	+	3,000,000[g]	1.3
Penthouse	Oct. 1985	"The War on Chiropractic"	Gary Null	++	3,770,000[g]	1.6
Penthouse	Nov. 1985	"Painful Treatment"	Gary Null	++	3,770,000[g]	1.6
Weight Watchers Magazine	Nov. 1985	"Should You Go to a Chiropractor?"	Sara Shapiro	++	Not listed	

CHIROPRACTIC ARTICLES (Continued)

Magazine	Date of Publication	Article Title	Author	Tone of Article	Circulation[a]	Percentage of U.S. Population Represented by Circulation[b]
Woman's World	Mar. 1986	"A New Life for Jeffrey" [in Precious Moments section]	Not given	++	Not listed	
Cosmopolitan	Mar. 1986	"Cosmo's Guide to Alternative Medicine"	Junius Adams	++	2,350,000[g]	1.0
New York	Mar. 10, 1986	"Oh, Your Aching Back"	Dava Sobel	+	430,841[g]	0.18
Harper's Bazaar		"Emotional Cool-Downs: New Relaxation Techniques"	Marilyn Boteler	++	600,000[g]	0.2
Prevention	May 1986	"A Fresh Look at Chiropractic Care"	Tom Shealey	++	2,821,501[g]	1.2
50 Plus	Sept. 1986	"Chiropractors: Taking a Crack at Hospitals"	David Diamond	+	290,000[g]	0.12
Prevention	Jan. 1987	"Chiropractic for Animals?"	Richard H. Pitcairn, D.V.M., Ph.D.	++	2,875,314[h]	1.2
Tennis	Feb. 1987	"Chiropractic: An Alternative Cure for Tennis Injuries"	Louise Ackerman	++	510,812[h]	0.2
Mademoiselle	June 1987	"Should You Trust the Touch of a Chiropractor?"	Laura Morice	+	1,236,392[h]	0.5
U.S. News & World Report	June 29, 1987	"Beyond the Limits of Traditional Medicine"	Lisa J. Moore	0	2,351,313[h]	1.0
World Tennis	Jan. 1988	"Hands That Heal"	Deborah Kleinman-Cindrich, D.C.	++	425,000[h]	0.2
Harvard Medical School Health Letter	Jan. 1988	"Low Back Pain: What about Chiropractors?"	Not given	0	300,000[f]	0.12

The Atlantic	Feb. 1988	"The Getting of Respect: American Chiropractors Are Still Fighting for Recognition from Medical Doctors"	Ellen Ruppel Shell	++	457,343[h]	0.18
Runner's World	Mar. 1988	"Advanced Injury Treatment: The Healing Touch"	Nelson Pena	+	425,000[i]	0.2
Prevention	Oct. 1989	"Inside Chiropractic: Exclusive Survey Results; How Americans Grade This Alternative-Healing Profession on Real-Life Results"	Gale Maleskey, ed.	+	2,850,000[i]	1.1

[a] Figures are from N.W. Ayer & Son's *American Newspaper Annual & Directory*, published yearly in Philadelphia. Precise figures come from sworn detailed statements made for the Audit Bureau of Circulations. Rounded figures are estimates. Circulation is defined by Ayer as "the average number of complete copies of all regular issues for a given period, exclusive of left over, unsold, returned, file, sample, exchange and advertisers' copies." (1921 ed., p. 6).

[b] Calculations are based on population figures for the appropriate year, taken from census data compiled in John M. Blum et al., *The National Experience*, 5th ed. (New York: Harcourt Brace Jovanovich, 1981), 920–22, and 7th ed. (1989), 864. Population figures for percentage calculations for 1988 and 1989 are taken from *Current Population Reports*, "Population Estimates and Projections."

[c] Figures are from Marietta Chicorel, ed., *Ulrich's International Periodicals Directory*, 12th ed. (New York: R.R. Bowker Co., 1967).

[d] Figures are from Merle Rohinsky, ed., *Ulrich's International Periodicals Directory*, 14th ed. (New York: R.R. Bowker Co., 1971).

[e] Figures from *Ulrich's*, 16th ed., 1975.

[f] Bill Katz and Linda Sternberg Katz, *Magazines for Libraries*, 4th ed. (New York: R.R. Bowker Co., 1982).

[g] Katz and Katz, *Magazines for Libraries*, 5th ed., 1986.

[h] Figures from *Ulrich's*, 27th ed., 1988–89.

[i] Katz and Katz, *Magazines for Libraries*, 6th ed., 1989.

Notes

Preface

1. See Theresa Gromala, " 'Bees in His Bonnet': D.D. Palmer's Students and Their Early Impact," *Chiropractic History* 6 (1986): 59. In the late nineteenth century, John Eric Erichsen was the leading authority on such "spinal concussion" and the injury became known as Erichsen's disease.

2. Judylaine Fine, *Conquering Back Pain: A Comprehensive Guide* (New York: Prentice Hall Press, 1987), 41–42. Even in the nineteenth century, some popular medical books began to recognize the potential problems of a sedentary life. William Buchan's extremely popular *[Domestic Medicine]: A Treatise on the Prevention and Cure of Diseases, by Regimen and Simple Medicines* (Cincinnati, 1841) (first published in Edinburgh in 1769 and printed and edited repeatedly in America) included advice for those engaged in "Desk Occupations."

3. W. H. Kirkaldy-Willis and J. D. Cassidy, "Spinal Manipulation in the Treatment of Low-Back Pain," *Canadian Family Physician* 31 (March 1985): 536; Fine, *Conquering Back Pain*, 10–11.

Chapter One. Subluxations, Science, and the Spine: D.D. Palmer and the Origins of Chiropractic

1. The complete advertisement is listed in Vern Gielow, *Old Dad Chiro: A Biography of D.D. Palmer, Founder of Chiropractic* (Davenport, Iowa: Bawden Bros., 1981), 44.

2. D.D. Palmer, *Text-Book of the Science, Art and Philosophy of Chiropractic, for Students and Practitioners* (Portland, Oreg.: Portland Printing House, 1910), 18. See also David D. Palmer, *The Palmers* (Davenport, Iowa: Bawden Bros., 1976), 77. David D. Palmer, known as Dave, was the grandson of D.D. Palmer and the son of Barlett Joshua (B.J.) Palmer.

3. The earliest seems to be an anonymous article entitled "New Pair of Ears" from March 1896. See Bobby Westbrooks, "The Troubled Legacy of Harvey Lillard: The Black Experience in Chiropractic," *Chiropractic History: The Archives and Journal of the Association for the History of Chiropractic*, 2 (1982): 47–48.

4. Palmer, *Science, Art and Philosophy of Chiropractic*, 18. The term *Chiropractic* (which means "done by hand") was suggested by a Palmer patient, the Reverend Samuel H. Weed, and adopted in January 1896. Curiously, the term serves as both an adjective and a noun.

Palmer's contention that spinal manipulation could cure deafness has been ridiculed frequently by orthodox medical practitioners and writers as an anatomical impossibility. See, for example, Morris Fishbein [M.D. and acting editor of the *Journal of the American Medical Association*], "Chiropractic," *American Mercury* (May 1925): 24–25, and Albert Q. Maisel, "Can Chiropractic Cure?" *Hygeia* (April 1946): 262. That the battle over this point still rages is illustrated by an announcement in the 1986 issue of *Chiropractic History*, a pro-chiropractic journal, which reported (p. 6) two recent medical studies (*The Chiropractic Report* by Dr. David Chapman-Smith and *Spinal Manipulation* by Dr. John Bourdillon) suggesting that manipulation of the spine can relieve deafness.

5. For a recitation of the conflicting accounts of the Lillard adjustment, see Gielow, *Old Dad Chiro*, 78–79. For discussion of the demand for "scientific medicine" in the 1890s, see Gerald E. Markowitz and David Rosner, "Doctors in Crisis: Medical Education and Medical Reform during the Progressive Era, 1895–1915," in *Health Care in America: Essays in Social History*, ed. Susan Reverby and David Rosner (Philadelphia: Temple University Press, 1979), esp. 187, 192. At the turn of the century, many respected medical authorities were arguing that drugs and chemicals would soon be alien to a truly scientific therapy. See Charles E. Rosenberg, "The Therapeutic Revolution: Medicine, Meaning, and Social Change in 19th-Century America," in *Sickness and Health in America: Readings in the History of Medicine and Public Health*, 2d ed., rev., ed. Judith Walzer Leavitt and Ronald L. Numbers (Madison: University of Wisconsin Press, 1985), esp. 48–49.

6. The entire article is quoted in Gielow, *Old Dad Chiro*, 65.

7. The *Moline Dispatch* article ("The Jury Couldn't Agree") and other local newspaper accounts concerning the case (such as "The Palmer-Wiltamuth Case" from the *Rock Island Union* and "Palmer Gets Judgment" from the *Davenport Times*) were clipped by Palmer and pasted in his August 13, 1890–February 13, 1892 daybook, photocopy housed in the Palmer College Library, Davenport, Iowa.

8. Palmer, *Science, Art and Philosophy of Chiropractic*, 17. For additional details on Port Perry and environs, see Gielow, *Old Dad Chiro*, 1–3, and Herbert K. Lee, "Portrait of Port Perry, Ontario, Birthplace of the Founder," *Chiropractic History* 5 (1985): 65–68.

9. Palmer, *Science, Art and Philosophy of Chiropractic*, 17.

10. Gielow, *Old Dad Chiro*, 4–5; Vern Gielow, "Daniel David Palmer: Rediscovering the Frontier Years, 1845–1887," *Chiropractic History* 1 (1981): 11.

11. Journal of D.D. Palmer, 1868–92, photocopy in the Palmer College Library. The journal is primarily a record of transactions from his various business ventures.

12. Perhaps more important in the long run to the spiritualist movement than the antics of the "rapping sisters" was the influence of Andrew Jackson Davis, the "Poughkeepsie Seer." A prolific writer, his harmonial philosophy (developed in *The Principles of Nature, Her Divine Revelation, and a Voice to Mankind* (1847), *The Great Harmonia* (1852), and subsequent writings) stressed the philosophic components of spiritualism and came increasingly into conflict with those who emphasized spirit phenomena. A full-scale rift between the two groups developed at the fourth national convention of the National Association of Spiritualists in 1867. See Robert W. Delp, "Andrew Jackson Davis: Prophet of American Spiritual-

ism," *Journal of American History* 54 (June 1967): 43–56. See also R. Laurence Moore, *In Search of White Crows* (New York: Oxford University Press, 1977). Although I have found no direct evidence that Palmer knew specifically of Andrew Jackson Davis, it is evident that Palmer sided with the philosophical spiritualists, disdaining the frolics of mediums.

13. The front and inside covers of the booklet are reproduced verbatim in Gielow, *Old Dad Chiro,* 24.

14. Hermeticism originated with the ancient Greek identification of Hermes with the Egyptian god, Thoth, the deity of wisdom and the scribe of the gods. A large body of Greek literature developed under the name Hermes Trismegistus, the "thrice great" Hermes, wisest of all and revered for his triple role as philosopher, priest, and king or lawgiver. The *corpus* included practical discourses (on astrology and the occult sciences and including recipes for the practice of astral magic) as well as a gnostic, philosophical *Hermetica.* Hermetic users of sympathetic magic operated on the premise that constant effluvia emanated from the stars toward earth and could be channeled by an operator who possessed the necessary knowledge. Each earthly object depended on occult sympathies poured down from its corresponding star. Everything in the universe was linked by a complex relationship of correspondences, and all were ultimately united because the All was One. By understanding the correspondences, the magician could enter and master the system. The magical art consisted of capturing and channeling the infusion of *spiritus* into *materia.* See the bibliographical essay for sources on the hermetic tradition.

15. Lester S. King, *The Philosophy of Medicine: The Early Eighteenth Century* (Cambridge: Harvard University Press, 1978), vi.

16. Ibid.

17. Ralph Waldo Trine, *In Tune with the Infinite or Fullness of Peace, Power, and Plenty,* originally published in 1897, quote from original preface. By the time of the Fiftieth Anniversary Edition (Indianapolis: Bobbs-Merrill, 1947), the book was a world classic and had sold more than a million and a quarter copies.

Harmonialism in America seems to be very similar in spirit to what German historians call "romantic medicine." See Iago Galdston, "Freud and Romantic Medicine," in *Freud: Modern Judgements,* ed. Frank Cioffi (London: Macmillan Press, 1973), 103–23.

18. Robert C. Fuller, *Alternative Medicine and American Religious Life* (New York: Oxford University Press, 1989), 35–36, 48. Fuller used Sylvester Graham as an example of the ascetic temperament and Emerson as an example of the aesthetic. Fuller also noted (p. 36) that harmonial healers involved with institutional Christianity tended to be less metaphysical than other harmonial types.

19. *Paracelsus: Selected Writings,* Bollingen Series, ed. Jolande Jacobi, trans. Norbert Guterman (New York: Pantheon, 1951), 140, 179–80. See also Walter Pagel, *Paracelsus: An Introduction to Philosophical Medicine in the Era of the Renaissance,* 2d rev. ed. (Basel: Karger, 1982), esp. 105–12.

20. Walter Pagel, *Joan Baptista Van Helmont: Reformer of Science and Medicine* (Cambridge: Cambridge University Press, 1982), 19, 96–129. See also Lynn Thorndike, *A History of Magic and Experimental Science,* 8 vols. (New York: Columbia University Press, 1923–58), 7: 218–40.

21. Maxwell's dates are obscure. The book was published by Georg Franck,

dean of the medical faculty at Heidelberg. See Thorndike, *History of Magic and Experimental Science,* 7: 229, 8: 419–21.

22. Frances A. Yates, *Giordano Bruno and the Hermetic Tradition* (Chicago: University of Chicago Press, 1964), 403–7, 440–47; Thorndike, *History of Magic and Experimental Science,* 7: 439–44. Fludd called his doctrines *pansophia,* a macro-microcosmical philosophy of universal harmonies, a term first used during the Renaissance by Platonic-Hermetic philosopher Francesco Patrizzi.

23. Yates, *Bruno and the Hermetic Tradition,* 60.

24. Thorndike, *History of Magic and Experimental Science,* 7: 301–2.

25. Herbert Butterfield, *The Origins of Modern Science, 1300–1800,* rev. ed. (New York: Free Press, 1957), 9–10.

26. Robert Darnton, *Mesmerism and the End of the Enlightenment in France* (Cambridge: Harvard University Press, 1968), 14, 3–4.

27. Gielow, *Old Dad Chiro,* 36.

28. Darnton, *Mesmerism,* vii, 10, 18, 20, 34, 36, 38–39, 157–58.

29. Ibid., 68–71. An English version of the report published in London in 1785 was entitled *Report of Dr. Benjamin Franklin and other commissioners, charged by the King of France with the examination of animal magnetism.* On the work of the commission and the subsequent turmoil, see Darnton, *Mesmerism,* 62–66.

30. See Joseph F. Kett, *The Formation of the American Medical Profession: The Role of Institutions, 1780–1860* (New Haven: Yale University Press, 1968), 144–45; Daniel N. Robinson, ed., *Significant Contributions to the History of Psychology, 1750–1920,* Series A, Orientations (Washington, D.C.: University Publications of America, 1977), 10: xxv–xxvi. A facsimile of Elliotson's work is printed in Robinson; included also is a fascimile of James Esdaile's *Mesmerism in India, and Its Practical Application in Surgery and Medicine* (London, 1846). Esdaile was influenced by Elliotson and also eschewed the spiritualist aspects of mesmerism.

The publisher's preface to the 1886 edition (orig. pub. 1847) of James Victor Wilson's *How to Magnetize, or Magnetism and Clairvoyance* (New York: Fowler & Wells), iii, noted the dulling effect of anesthetics on the use of animal magnetism in surgery.

31. Eric T. Carlson, "Charles Poyen Brings Mesmerism to America," *Journal of the History of Medicine and Allied Sciences* 15 (April 1960): 121–32. Poyen himself viewed animal magnetism as a branch of natural science (p. 124).

32. An example of this popularization of mesmeric concepts is a long portion in the 1851 domestic medical guide of American physician Frederick Hollick, *The Family Physician; or, the True Art of Healing the Sick in All Diseases Whatever,* 91–123. Hollick discussed the magnetic experiments of German chemist Baron Charles von Reichenbach (who had influenced Elliotson) and gushed in wonder (p. 93) over "that subtile power which pervades the whole universe."

33. The complete obituary is reprinted in Gielow, *Old Dad Chiro,* 38–40, presumably from the *Ottumwa Democrat.* Joseph E. Maynard, D.C., Ph.C. [Philosopher of Chiropractic], *Healing Hands: The Story of the Palmer Family, Discoverers and Developers of Chiropractic,* rev. ed. (Mobile, Ala.: Jonorm Publishers, 1977) claimed that Palmer was actually a student of Caster's and reported a conversation between the two (pp. 9–10). Maynard's book, however, is an anecdotal

history written in such a folksy, homespun style that a healthy skepticism concerning detail is warranted. It *is* safe to assume that Palmer at least knew of Caster's work.

34. Gielow, *Old Dad Chiro*, 40–44; Gielow, "Daniel David Palmer: Frontier Years," 12.

35. n.p., n.d., pp. 6–7, in *D.D. Palmer's Portable Library*, photocopy of books owned by Palmer, bound by Palmer College Library, 1982. See also E.D. Babbitt, *Vital Magnetism: The Life Fountain* (New York: by the author, n.d.), 16 (also in *Palmer's Portable Library*) for a similar explanation that faith in the magnetist was helpful but not necessary.

36. Babbitt, *Vital Magnetism*, 26–28, 109.

37. The other titles in the *Portable Library* are *The Moral Aphorisms and Terseological Teachings of Confucius* (Battle Creek, Mich.: 1870); *Be Thyself: A Discourse.* (Boston, n.d.); *The Deluge in the Light of Modern Science: A Discourse.* (Boston: 1872); *A Lecture on the Evolution of Life in Earth and Spirit Conditions* (Milwaukee: 1882); *Diana: A Psycho-Fyziological Essay on Sexual Relations, For Married Men and Women*, 3d ed., rev. and enl. (New York: Burnz & Co., 1885); *Cupid's Yokes: Or the Binding Forces of Conjugal Life* (Princeton: Co-operative Publishing Co., n.d.).

38. For discussion of the rural attitude toward education, see Richard Hofstadter, *Anti-intellectualism in American Life* (New York: Alfred A. Knopf, 1963), 277–80. Earlier in the century, Samuel Thomson had used his lack of education as a boon to selling his botanic program by emphasizing his work as a calling. See Martin Kaufman, *Homeopathy in America: The Rise and Fall of a Medical Heresy* (Baltimore: Johns Hopkins University Press, 1971), 18–19. Thomson also believed that formal medical education was unnecessary and even dangerous. William G. Rothstein, *American Physicians in the Nineteenth Century: From Sects to Science* (Baltimore: Johns Hopkins University Press, 1972), 143.

On the McAnnulty rule, see James Harvey Young, *The Medical Messiahs: A Social History of Health Quackery in Twentieth-Century America* (Princeton: Princeton University Press, 1967), 69–73.

39. D.D. Palmer's daybooks. See also Gielow, *Old Dad Chiro*, 52–53, for the partial text of a Palmer advertisement; pp. 57–58 for the text of a newspaper article in the What Cheer *Patriot* (n.d.), which gives some details of Palmer's practice; and p. 59 for a year-by-year listing of Palmer's cash receipts. The Palmer daybooks also list debts he still hoped to collect. Figures for average physician income are from Paul Starr, *The Social Transformation of American Medicine* (New York: Basic Books, 1982), 84–85. Virginia G. Drachman, "Female Solidarity and Professional Success: The Dilemma of Women Doctors in Late 19th-Century America," in *Sickness and Health in America*, notes (p. 175) that the average annual income for *women* doctors in 1881 was $3,000.

40. Palmer, *Science, Art and Philosophy of Chiropractic*, 111, 128.

41. *Hippocratic Writings*, trans. Francis Adams, Great Books of the Western World, vol. 10 (Chicago: Encyclopedia Britannica, 1952), 95, 128–29; Marcus Bach, *The Chiropractic Story* (Austell, Ga.: Si-Nel Publishing & Sales Co., 1968), 246.

42. Erwin H. Ackerknecht, *Therapeutics from the Primitives to the 20th Century*

(New York: Hafner Press, 1973), 28–29. Ackerknecht considers him to be "the precursor of certain modern physiotherapeutic sects."

43. James F. Ransom, "The Origins of Chiropractic Physiological Therapeutics: Howard, Forester and Schulze," *Chiropractic History* 4 (1984): 47.

44. Robert T. Anderson, "On Doctors and Bonesetters in the 16th and 17th Centuries," *Chiropractic History* 3 (1983): 11–14. Sarah Mapp is mentioned in *Chiropractic in New Zealand: Report of the Commission of Inquiry* (Wellington, New Zealand: 1979; reprint ed., Davenport, Iowa: Palmer College of Chiropractic, n.d.), 37, and in Marshall Smith, "If Your Back Is Out, You're 'In,' " *Life*, April 9, 1965, p. 71.

45. The long title of the book is *The Compleat Bone-setter, wherein the Method of Curing Broken Bones and Strains and Dislocated Joynts, together with Ruptures, commonly called Broken Bellies, is fully demonstrated.* Only three copies of the first edition are extant. Robert J.T. Joy, "The Natural Bonesetters with Special Reference to the Sweet Family of Rhode Island: A Study of an Early Phase of Orthopedics," *Bulletin of the History of Medicine* 20 (September–October 1954): 416–18; Anderson, "On Doctors and Bonesetters," 12.

46. Joy, "The Natural Bonesetters," 416; Anderson, "On Doctors and Bonesetters," 12–13.

47. This particular medical critique is from Sir James Paget, "Clinical Lectures on Cases That Bonesetters Cure," *British Medical Journal* 1 (1867): 1, quoted in Joy, "The Natural Bonesetters," 420.

48. J.B. Brown, *Reports of Cases in the Boston Orthopedic Institution* (Boston: D. Clapp, 1844), 1, quoted in Joy, "The Natural Bonesetters," 424. In the traditional medical view, specialization of any type meant quackery; treatment of a specific illness with a specific drug was also suspect. See John Duffy, *The Healers: A History of American Medicine* (Urbana: University of Illinois Press, 1976), 250; Rothstein, *American Physicians in the Nineteenth Century*, 207–16; Rosenberg, "The Therapeutic Revolution," 42.

49. Joy, "The Natural Bonesetters," 429. Job Sweet's work with the French and the Burr incident are also mentioned by D.D. Palmer in *The Science, Art and Philosophy of Chiropractic*, 547.

50. Cited in Duffy, *The Healers*, 123.

51. Palmer, *Science, Art and Philosophy of Chiropractic*, 544–45.

52. Ibid., 549.

53. Norman Gevitz, *The D.O.'s: Osteopathic Medicine in America* (Baltimore: Johns Hopkins University Press, 1982), 15–17.

54. Palmer's claim that he was never in Kirksville is in *Science, Art and Philosophy of Chiropractic*, 391–92. For countervailing evidence, see Russell W. Gibbons, "The Evolution of Chiropractic: Medical and Social Protest in America," in *Modern Developments in the Principles and Practice of Chiropractic*, ed. Scott Haldeman (New York: Appleton-Century-Crofts, 1980), 13. See also Gielow, *Old Dad Chiro*, 139 n.2, and James W. Brantingham, "Still and Palmer: The Impact of the First Osteopath and the First Chiropractor," *Chiropractic History* 6 (1986): 19–22. For an anecdotal account of a supposed debate between Palmer and Still, see L. Ted Frigard, "Clinton, Iowa c. 1906(?) 'The Old Doctor' vs. 'Old Dad Chiro,' " *Chiropractic History* 7 (December 1987): 6–7.

55. Palmer, *Science, Art and Philosophy of Chiropractic,* 139.

56. *Chiropractic in New Zealand,* 40; Palmer, *Science, Art and Philosophy of Chiropractic,* 128, 141–42, 810, 974. See also pp. 389–92 for statements by osteopaths citing differences between osteopathy and chiropractic. For an early and uncharacteristically balanced article that finds differences between osteopathy and chiropractic, see Channing Frothingham, "Osteopathy, Chiropractic, and the Profession of Medicine," *Atlantic Monthly* (July 1922): 75–81.

57. Palmer, *Science, Art and Philosophy of Chiropractic,* 491–93, 399, 496. See Maynard, *Healing Hands,* 207, for elaboration on the sunbeam metaphor. For Palmer, *nature* was an inadequate term for Innate because "nature takes in the universe whereas I wanted a term to express individuality" (*Science, Art and Philosophy,* 492, cf. 501). "Mind," however, was too restrictive: "Innate is not the mind. Innate is the intelligence back of and controller of the mind as well as of every thought. . . . Mind is a product of Innate" (p. 362). On p. 616, in apparent contradiction, Palmer wrote that "Mind is a production of Educated." This problem could perhaps be reconciled by elaborating a distinction between *product* and *production,* but Palmer failed to do so.

58. Palmer, *Science, Art and Philosophy of Chiropractic,* 494–95.

59. Ibid., pp. 499, 486, 19.

60. Palmer defined *nerve force* as "the energy expressed by the nervous system in performing any of the functions," the "power expended in performing the various acts of the body." Ibid., 484.

61. See Duffy, *The Healers,* 183, for the idea that medical men were losing faith in the possibility of discovering a grand principle.

62. Stephen Nissenbaum, *Sex, Diet, and Debility in Jacksonian America: Sylvester Graham and Health Reform* (Westport, Conn.: Greenwood Press, 1980), 54–57; George W. Corner, ed., *The Autobiography of Benjamin Rush: His "Travels through Life" Together with His Commonplace Book for 1789–1813* (Princeton: Princeton University Press, 1948), Appendix 1, 361–66. Even though Rush's heroic measures stand on the opposite end of the therapeutic spectrum from Palmer's drugless approach, both embraced the notion of a single cause of disease. Perhaps the most curious monism of all was the theory of eighteenth-century British doctor James Graham, who held that all diseases came from wearing too much clothing. See William L. Whitwell, "James Graham: Master Quack," *Journal of Eighteenth Century Life* 4 (December 1977): 43–49.

63. Starr, *Social Transformation of American Medicine,* 54–59. In the 1820s and 1830s, Americans who studied in Paris typically adopted the therapeutic skepticism of the French, which began to erode the monistic approach to disease.

64. John Higham, "The Reorientation of American Culture in the 1890's," in *The Origins of Modern Consciousness,* ed. John Weiss (Detroit: Wayne State University Press, 1965), 35, 27.

65. According to Joseph Maynard (*Healing Hands,* 85–86), B.J. Palmer met Macfadden at the Mardi Gras in New Orleans (n.d.). B.J. advised Macfadden to quit his one-man traveling show and put his energies into publishing, a venture that made Macfadden a fortune. Maynard noted that the two met "on various occasions" over the years. B.J. once featured Macfadden on an athletic float in a lyceum parade in Davenport.

Macfadden became a vigorous supporter of chiropractic. In 1922, Macfadden wrote to Nathan L. Miller, governor of New York, requesting a veto of the Bloomfield-Lattin Bill #1440, an antichiropractic bill designed to banish chiropractic from the state. "I have used chiropractic for a number of years," Macfadden wrote Miller, "and literally hundreds of thousands of the citizens of this State have been making use of it to their distinct benefit." Macfadden to Miller, n.d., Lyndon Lee Papers, Misc. Material: Special Correspondence, Palmer College Archives, Davenport, Iowa.

CHAPTER TWO. OF DOCTOR BOOKS, ANODYNES, AND "OLD STUBBORN PAINS IN THE BACK" IN NINETEENTH-CENTURY AMERICA

1. James Parkinson, *The Town and Country Friend and Physician; or, An Affectionate Address on the Preservation of Health, and the Removal of Disease on its First Appearance; Supposed to be Delivered by a Country Physician to the Circle of his Friends and Patients on his Retiring from Business: with Cursory Observations on the Treatment of Children, etc. Intended for the Promotion of Domestic Happiness* (Philadelphia: James Humphreys, 1803), 74–75. Ward quoted in William Barlow and David Powell, "Malthus A. Ward, Frontier Physician, 1815–1823," *Journal of the History of Medicine and Allied Sciences* 32 (1977): 290.

2. John Tennent, *Every Man his own Doctor: or, the Poor Planter's Physician. Prescribing, Plain and Easy Means for Persons to cure themselves of all, or most of the Distempers, incident to this Climate, and with very little Charge, the Medicines being chiefly of the Growth and Production of this Country,* 4th ed. (Philadelphia, 1736), frontispiece. Frank Luther Mott in *Golden Multitudes: The Story of Best Sellers in the United States* (New York: Macmillan, 1947), 301, placed the original publication date as 1734, almost certainly a mistake, since a fourth edition was printed in 1736. In addition, the *Dictionary of American Medical Biography* (Westport, Conn.: Greenwood Press, 1984), 735, placed the publication date of the *second* edition in 1724. It seems likely then, that the book was published originally sometime in the second decade of the century. For a brief description of Tennent's often "unhappy and scandalous" life, see *Dictionary of American Medical Biography,* 734–35.

3. Charles E. Rosenberg, "Medical Text and Social Context: Explaining William Buchan's *Domestic Medicine," Bulletin of the History of Medicine* 57 (Spring 1983): 22–42. According to Rosenberg, there were at least 142 English language versions. Claxton of Philadelphia published the last American version in 1871 (p. 22, n. 1). There was an American reprint of the book as early as 1772 (p. 41); Mott, *Golden Multitudes,* 301; Martin Kaufman, " 'Step Right Up, Ladies and Gentlemen . . . ': Patent Medicines in 19th-Century America," in Robert James Maddox, ed., *Annual Editions: American History,* 7th ed. (Guilford, Conn.: Dushkin, 1983), vol. 1, *Pre-colonial through Reconstruction,* 147–48.

4. Mott, *Golden Multitudes,* 301.

5. *New York Courier,* n.d., quoted in Ray Vaughn Pierce, *The People's Common Sense Medical Adviser in Plain English; Or, Medicine Simplified,* 69th ed. [?] (Buffalo, N.Y.: World's Dispensary Printing Office, 1895), 909.

6. *The Buffalo Commercial,* n.d., quoted in Pierce, *People's Common Sense*

Medical Adviser, 908. Such beaming, self-serving statements were often reprinted in testimonial form in the various doctor books.

7. Ibid., 869–70.

8. Thomas Jefferson to James Ewell, March 1, 1808, quoted in James Ewell, *The Medical Companion, or Family Physician,* 6th ed. (Baltimore: 1822), vi.

9. Ibid., 789–92. For domestic medicine chests as an extension of orthodox practice, see J. K. Crellin, "Domestic Medicine Chests: Microcosms of 18th and 19th-Century Medical Practice," *Pharmacy in History* 21 (1979): 122–31.

10. J. A. Brown, *The Family Guide to Health* (Providence, R.I.: 1837), 211–15, 221.

11. William Daily, *The Indian Doctor's Practice of Medicine. Daily's Family Physician: Important to Every One! Health the Poor Man's Riches!—The Rich Man's Bliss! Giving the Symptoms of Diseases, and a Vegetable Treatment of the Diseases of Men, Women, and Children* (Louisville, Ky.: 1848), 209–10.

12. John George Hohman, *The Long Lost Friend or Faithful & Christian Instructions Containing Wondrous and Well-Tried Arts & Remedies, for Man as Well as Animals* (Harrisburg, Pa.: 1850), 8.

13. William M. Hand, *The House Surgeon and Physician; Designed To-Assist Heads of Families, Travellers, and Sea-Faring People, in Discerning, Distinguishing, and Curing Diseases; with Concise Directions for the Preparation and Use of a Numerous Collection of The Best American Remedies: Together With Many of the Most Approved, from the Shop of the Apothecary. All in Plain English* (New Haven, Conn.: Silus Andrus, 1820), xi.

14. *New York Medical Repository* (n.p., n.d.), quoted in Ewell, *The Medical Companion,* vii. J. Cam Massie in *Treatise on the Eclectic Southern Practice of Medicine* (Philadelphia: Thomas, Cowperthwait & Co., 1854), 7, noted that works of domestic medicine had "deluged the country."

15. For the development of aspirin and its usage, see K. D. Rainsford, *Aspirin and the Salicylates* (London: Butterworths, 1984), esp. chap. 1; Marie Harvin, comp., "Acetylsalicylic Acid, the Story of Aspirin: Notes to Accompany an Exhibit at the National Library of Medicine," Washington, 1959, (typescript). G. Motherby, in *A New Medical Dictionary, or General Repository of Physic,* 5th ed. (London: S. Hamilton, 1801), 88, defined anodynes as "medicines which ease pain, and procure sleep" and divided them into three types—paregorics, which "assuage pain"; hypnotics, which relieve pain by inducing sleep; and narcotics, which "ease the patient by stupifying him." According to Motherby, by the early nineteenth century the term *anodyne* was "generally employed for those means only which relieve pain by diminishing or destroying sensibility."

16. Thomas Thacher, *A Brief Rule to guide the Common-People of New-England how to order themselves and theirs in the Small Pocks, or Measels* (Boston, 1677; facsimile ed., Baltimore: Johns Hopkins University Press, 1937), xiii, 6.

17. Duffy, *The Healers,* 41. For a discussion of the "omnipresent preacher-physician" in colonial America, see pp. 34–41.

18. C. Wayne Callaway, "John Wesley's *Primitive Physick:* An Essay in Appreciation," *Mayo Clinic Proceedings* 49 (May 1974): 318–24; Samuel J. Rogal, "Pills for the Poor: John Wesley's *Primitive Physick,*" *The Yale Journal of Biology and*

Medicine 51 (January–February 1978): 81–90; Nissenbaum, *Sex, Diet, and Debility*, 43.

19. John Wesley, *Primitive Physick: or, an Easy and Natural Method of Curing Most Diseases*, 14th ed. (Philadelphia, 1770), 57.

20. Ibid., 61–62.

21. Ibid., 63–64.

22. See Duffy, *The Healers*, 41.

23. Wesley, *Primitive Physick*, xvii.

24. Tennent, *Every Man His Own Doctor*, 50–51.

25. Rosenberg, "Medical Text and Social Context," 29–30.

26. For the development of opium use in the United States, see Joseph L. Zentner, "Opiate Use in America during the Eighteenth and Nineteenth Centuries: Origins of a Modern Scourge," *Studies in History and Society* 5 (1974): 40–54, and Rothstein, *American Physicians in the Nineteenth Century*, 109–94.

27. John C. Gunn, *Gunn's Domestic Medicine, or Poor Man's Friend, in the Hours of Affliction, Pain, and Sickness* (n.p.: B. J. Webb & Bro., 1840), 697–99.

28. Edward Kremers and George Urdang, *History of Pharmacy: A Guide and a Survey*, 2d ed., rev. and enl. (Philadelphia: J. B. Lippincott, 1951), 529.

29. Gunn, *Gunn's Domestic Medicine*, 697–98.

30. See, for example, Hand, *The House Surgeon and Physician*, 51, and Alexander Thomson, *The Family Physician; or, Domestic Medical Friend: containing Plain and Practical Instructions for the Prevention and Cure of diseases, According to the newest Improvements and Discoveries, with a series of chapters on Collateral subjects; comprising every thing relative to the Theory and Principles of the Medical Art, necessary to be known by the Private Practitioner. The Whole Adapted to the use of those heads of families who have not had a classical or medical education* (New York: James Oram, 1802), 410–12.

31. See Samuel Thomson, *A Narrative of the Life and Medical Discoveries of Samuel Thomson: containing an account of his System of Practice and the manner of curing disease with Vegetable Medicine, upon a plan entirely new; to which is prefixed an introduction to his New Guide to Health or Botanic Family Physician; containing the principle upon which the system is founded, with remarks on fever, steaming, poison, etc.*, 8th ed. (Columbus, Ohio: 1832), esp. 41–51; Kaufman, *Homeopathy in America*. For domestic medical guides penned by practitioners of alternative medical sects, see Ronald L. Numbers, "Do-It-Yourself the Sectarian Way," in *"Send Us a Lady Physician:" Women Doctors in America, 1835–1920*, ed. Ruth J. Abram (New York: W. W. Norton, 1985), 43–54.

32. Starr, *Social Transformation of American Medicine*, 42; James Harvey Young, *The Toadstool Millionaires: A Social History of Patent Medicines in America before Federal Regulation* (Princeton: Princeton University Press, 1961), 36–37. On the yellow fever epidemic, see J. H. Powell, *Bring Out Your Dead: The Great Plague of Yellow Fever in Philadelphia in 1793* (Philadelphia: University of Pennsylvania Press, 1949), and Martin S. Pernick, "Politics, Parties, and Pestilence: Epidemic Yellow Fever in Philadelphia and the Rise of the First Party System," in *Sickness and Health in America: Readings in the History of Medicine and Public Health*, 2d ed., rev., eds. Judith Walzer Leavitt and Ronald L. Numbers (Madison: University of Wisconsin Press, 1985), 356–71.

33. Rosenberg, "The Therapeutic Revolution," 40–41; see also Rosenberg, "Medical Text and Social Context," 31–35.

34. William M. Hand (*The House Surgeon and Physician*, 32) even prescribed bleeding the patient for a dislocation. The logic was that loss of blood would lead to unconsciousness, relaxing the patient and making manipulation much easier. See also Benjamin Rush, *Medical Inquiries and Observations*, 3d ed. (Philadelphia: 1809), 4: 378–79, cited by Kaufman, *Homeopathy in America*, 7.

35. The material from Thomson's *Family Physician* is from pp. 317–21 and 272–75 passim.

36. On dry-cupping, see Thomson, *Family Physician*, 320.

37. Ewell, *The Medical Companion*, 609–10. Concoctions with both internal and external uses were common.

38. Brown, *The Family Guide to Health*, 208, 210.

39. For additional examples, see *Every Man's Doctor: or Family Guide to Health, Containing a Condensed Description of the Various Causes and Symptoms of Diseases with an Appendix, Showing the Medical Properties of the Most Valuable Roots and Herbs to Which is Added 150 Recipes* (New York: J. K. Wellman, 1845), 44–45, 55, 59; Hand, *The House Surgeon and Physician*, 43; Daily, *Indian Doctor's Practice of Medicine*, 57, 61, 169; Massie, *Eclectic Southern Practice of Medicine*, 191–200; Isaac Shinn, *The Ready Advisor and Family Guide: A New Compilation of Valuable Recipes and Guides to Health* (Chicago: Church & Goodman, 1866), 107; Henry Rice Stout, *Our Family Physician: A Plain, Practical and Reliable Guide to the Direction and Treatment of all the Diseases Common to this Country* (Peoria, Ill.: 1887), 450–51; John King, *The American Family Physician; or, Domestic Guide to Health. Prepared Expressly for the use of Families, in Language Adapted to the Understanding of the People. Arranged in Two Divisions* (Indianapolis: Robert Douglass, 1892), 323–28, Division II, pp. 149–51.

40. Kathryn Kish Sklar, *Catharine Beecher: A Study in American Domesticity* (New York: W. W. Norton, 1973), 205–8; Duffy, *The Healers*, 121–22.

41. For an assessment of medical complaints peculiar to women, see Sarah Stage, *Female Complaints: Lydia Pinkham and the Business of Women's Medicine* (New York: W. W. Norton, 1979).

42. John S. Haller, Jr., and Robin M. Haller, *The Physician and Sexuality in Victorian America* (Urbana: University of Illinois Press, 1974), 31–32, 168, 170.

43. Sklar, *Catharine Beecher*, 205; Catharine E. Beecher, *Letters to the People on Health and Happiness* (New York: Harper & Brothers, 1855; repr. ed., New York: Arno Press, 1972), appendix, p. 10.

44. Massie, *Eclectic Southern Practice of Medicine*, 37–39.

45. See Duffy, *The Healers*, 122.

46. Haller and Haller, *Physician and Sexuality*, 5–10; Barbara Sicherman, "The Uses of a Diagnosis: Doctors, Patients, and Neurasthenia," in *Sickness and Health in America*, 22–35. For detailed discussion of the researches of Emil du Bois-Reymond and others which provided an underpinning for the views and practices of American physicians, see E. G. T. Liddell, *The Discovery of Reflexes* (Oxford: Clarendon Press, 1960), esp. 31–47.

47. Haller and Haller, *Physician and Sexuality*, 11–15.

48. Frederick Hollick, *The Family Physician; or, the True Art of Healing the*

Sick in All Diseases Whatever (Philadelphia: T. B. Peterson, 1851), 151, 160, chap. 6 passim.

49. Shinn, *Ready Advisor and Family Guide*, 110–11.

50. George M. Beard, *Our Home Physician: A New and Popular Guide to the Art of Preserving Health and Treating Disease; with Plain Advice for all the Medical and Surgical Emergencies of the Family* (New York: E. B. Treat & Co., 1869), 485–86.

51. Ibid., 485–86, 790, 847, 989, 1011.

52. *Harper's Weekly*, October 29, 1881, facsimile in Haller and Haller, *Physician and Sexuality*, 155. In the June 15, 1889, issue, *Harper's Weekly* also advertised for home use the "Dr. Huber Electro-Magnetic Dry Cell Pocket Medical Battery," which furnished "4000 Electro-Magnetic Vibrations" per minute and promised to cure, among other ailments, neuralgia, lumbago, and nervous debility. See facsimile in Haller and Haller, p. 20.

53. Pierce, *People's Common Sense Medical Advisor*, 887, 879–82. For another doctor book with gadgets prominently displayed, see John Harvey Kellogg, *The Home Book of Medicine: A Family Guide in Health and Disease* (Battle Creek, Mich.: Modern Medicine Publishing Co., 1906), esp. 1460–63, which displays devices designed specifically to straighten curvature of the spine. On the electrical "gadget boom," see James Harvey Young, *The Medical Messiahs: A Social History of Health Quackery in Twentieth-Century America* (Princeton: Princeton University Press, 1967), 239–59.

54. Walter Rauschenbusch, *Christianizing the Social Order* (New York: Macmillan, 1912), 248–49.

55. For discussion of the therapeutic value of human touch, see Merrijoy Kelner, Oswald Hall, and Ian Coulter, *Chiropractors: Do They Help? A Study of Their Education and Practice* (Toronto: Fitzhenry & Whiteside, 1980), 8–15. For a late nineteenth-century doctor book that touted message as "a new method of healing" and provided the reader with home lessons in back message for "rheumatism, backache, paralysis, nervousness and spinal trouble," see B. G. Jefferis and J. L. Nichols, *The Household Guide or Domestic Cyclopedia. A Practical Family Physician. Home Remedies and Home Treatment on All Diseases. An Instructor on Nursing, Housekeeping and Home Adornments*, 19th ed. (Atlanta: J. L. Nichols & Co., 1897), 192–95.

56. Hollick, *The Family Physician*, 161–62; King, *The American Family Physician*, Division II, pp. 151–53.

57. Euphoria over the long-term value of electromagnetic treatments had waned by the turn of the century. See King, *The American Family Physician*, Division I, p. 326. The rest cure suggested by King (Division II, p. 153) was a passive treatment unlikely to impress the back sufferer.

58. Pierce, *People's Common Sense Medical Adviser*, 431–32.

CHAPTER THREE. THE CHIROPRACTIC KALEIDOSCOPE

1. As Vern Gielow explained in *Old Dad Chiro*, 140 n.1, "congestion of the brain" was a generic term covering a number of conditions ranging from ringing in the ears to arteriosclerosis to massive cerebral problems.

Verbatim transcriptions of two counts against B.J. from the Scott County, Iowa, records are given in Gielow, *Old Dad Chiro*, 125–26.

2. Two paeans to B.J. contended that D.D. was also lecturing at Universal Chiropractic College. See Maynard, *Healing Hands*, 73, and A. August Dye, *The Evolution of Chiropractic: Its Discovery and Development* (Philadelphia: by the author, 1421 Arch Street, 1939), 49. Gielow, generally more balanced in his account, did not mention this in *Old Dad Chiro*.

3. A rumor developed that Palmer was taken unconscious to a local hospital. Chittenden Turner, *The Rise of Chiropractic* (Los Angeles: Powell Publishing Co., 1931), 32, presented this as fact. It is, however, almost surely false. Gielow mentioned nothing about a hospital stay. Maynard (*Healing Hands*, 74) reported D.D. phoning "a friend" from his room at B.J.'s house (where he almost surely *was* staying) with news that his son had tried to kill him with a car. Maynard then labeled the charge a lie, the result of a "mentally unbalanced" mind generated by bitterness and hatred. All of these accounts must be approached cautiously.

4. Gielow, *Old Dad Chiro*, 123–28; *The Davenport Democrat and Leader*, December 28, 1914, and *The Davenport Times*, December 28, 1914, facsimiles printed in Maynard, *Healing Hands*, 82.

5. Lyndon E. Lee, "For several years past . . . ," Lyndon Lee Papers, Misc. Manuscripts: Folder #1, Palmer College Archives, Davenport, Iowa; Gielow, *Old Dad Chiro*, 81, 90; Harry Gallaher, *History of Chiropractic: A History of the Philosophy, Art and Science of Chiropractic and Chiropractors in Oklahoma Together with a Biographical History of the Prominent Exponents of the Science in Oklahoma* (Guthrie, Okla.: William E. Welch and William H. Pattie, 1930), 30; Russell W. Gibbons, "The Rise of the Chiropractic Educational Establishment, 1897–1980," in *Who's Who in Chiropractic*, 2d ed., ed. Fern Lints-Dzaman (Littleton, Colo.: Who's Who in Chiropractic International Publishing Co., 1980), 340.

According to Maynard (*Healing Hands*, 12), D.D. frequently beat his children and on occasion was arrested and locked up overnight. Maynard claimed that B.J. suffered a fractured vertebra and curvature of the spine because of the beatings. In the introduction to B.J.'s *The Bigness of the Fellow Within* (Davenport, Iowa: Palmer Chiropractic Fountain Head, 1949), v, Palmer School Dean Herbert C. Hender claimed that B.J. was often forced to sleep in dry-goods boxes in subfreezing alleys.

6. Oakley Smith, *Naprapathic Genetics: Being a Study of the Origin and Development of Naprapathy*, 2 vols. ([Chicago]: by the author, 1932), 1:6.

7. Gielow, *Old Dad Chiro*, 96–98; Gibbons, "Rise of the Chiropractic Educational Establishment," 340–42; Turner, *Rise of Chiropractic*, 26–27; Dye, *Evolution of Chiropractic*, 17, 286. D.D. Palmer mentioned a clinic he held in Santa Barbara, California, on July 1, 1903, where he "discovered" that the body was heated by nerves and not by blood. See *Science, Art and Philosophy of Chiropractic*, 485.

Exactly when D.D. returned to Davenport is unclear, but his indictment for practicing medicine without a license in 1906 dates his offense from "on or about the first day of December, 1904."

8. "A Letter Written to S.M. Langworthy, D.C., By D.D. Palmer When He Was Confined In The Scott County Jail, April, 1906," *The Chiropractor, A Monthly Journal* 2 (April–May 1906), reprinted in B.J. Palmer, *History Repeats* (Davenport, Iowa: Chiropractic Fountain Head, 1951), 69–71.

9. Gielow, *Old Dad Chiro,* 103–14, is a virtual scrapbook for the case. He included verbatim transcriptions of the charge against Palmer and numerous newspaper articles about the case in *The Davenport Democrat and Leader,* as well as articles written by Palmer for the paper, including an April 6 piece, "How to be Happy in Jail: Dr. D.D. Palmer Writes a New Line of Valuable Maxims. From the County Jail He Sends Messages of Optimism to the Outside World," and another entitled "Chiropractic Sunbeams," in which Palmer described himself as a persecuted scientist, the victim of a corrupt medical establishment.

Maynard (*Healing Hands,* 41, 43) stated that B.J. was indicted at the same time as his father but never stood trial. Walter R. Rhodes in *The Official History of Chiropractic in Texas* (Austin: Texas Chiropractic Association, 1978), 24–25, also made the same assertion. They were probably confusing an earlier indictment against B.J. (April 16, 1903, which apparently never was tried) with the 1906 incident. Maynard, especially, was frequently in error regarding detail, and his "facts" should not be accepted uncritically.

10. Verbatim transcriptions of the arbitration report and D.D.'s receipt are given in Dye, *Evolution of Chiropractic,* 19. See also Gielow, *Old Dad Chiro,* 115–16; Rhodes, *Chiropractic in Texas,* 24–26; Maynard, *Healing Hands,* 44–45. The restless Palmer also reentered the school business, establishing a string of short-lived institutions and partnerships—the Palmer-Gregory College of Chiropractic in Oklahoma City with Alva A. Gregory; the Fountain Head School also in Oklahoma City; the Pacific Chiropractic College (a predecessor of Western States College) in Portland, Oregon, with John LaValley; and a solo venture that failed, the D.D. Palmer School of Chiropractic.

11. Palmer, *Science, Art and Philosophy of Chiropractic,* 425–26, 485, 819. On p. 507, Palmer quoted a bulletin from the Palmer School written by B.J., which described his son's position.

12. The pamphlet is reprinted in Gielow, *Old Dad Chiro,* 93–94; cf. [Howard A. Thomas], "Topical Index of Lerner's Reports on the History of Chiropractic," entry for vol. 2, pp. 119–35, Lee Papers, Correspondence 1955–76, Palmer College Archives, Davenport, Iowa.

13. In *Science, Art and Philosophy of Chiropractic,* 641, D.D. mentioned an article on "Innate Intelligence" he wrote "over six years ago," placing it in 1904; cf. Joseph Donahue, "D.D. Palmer and Innate Intelligence: Development, Division and Derision," *Chiropractic History* 6 (1986): 31.

14. "Immortality" is reprinted in B.J. Palmer's *History Repeats,* 65–68.

15. [Thomas], "Topical Index of Lerner's Reports," entry for vol. 7, pp. 604–60, Lee Papers, Palmer College Archives; William S. Rehm, "Legally Defensible: Chiropractic in the Courtroom and After, 1907," *Chiropractic History* 6 (1986): 51–55. Rehm was mistaken (p. 54) in his contention that D.D. had dealt originally only in the "structure of the body." Rehm took D.D.'s mechanical aberration as a primary position and failed to understand his harmonial background.

In the wake of the Morikubo case, chiropractic "philosophy" provided a useful legal defense for distinguishing chiropractic from osteopathy and from the medical profession.

16. For epithets, see Dye, *Evolution of Chiropractic,* 47, 54, 92, 127, 151, and Russell W. Gibbons, "Forgotten Parameters [*sic*] of General Practice: The

Chiropractic Obstetrician," *Chiropractic History* 2 (1982): 30. Turner, *Rise of Chiropractic,* 280–81, emphasized the practical and business-minded approach of B.J.; cf. Dye, *Evolution of Chiropractic,* 16–18. See reproductions of "Chiropractic zingers," *Chiropractic History* 3 (1983): 24, for a facsimile of a Palmer advertisement that declared: "Mixing is Failing. Mixers are Failures, To Mix is to Fail."

17. Dye (*Evolution of Chiropractic,* 113–53), a disciple of B.J., provided an extended discussion of the straight/mixer split.

18. Willard Carver's Personal Diary, p. 11, Logan College of Chiropractic Archives, Chesterfield, Mo.

19. See *Who's Who in Chiropractic,* 2d ed., s.v. "Carver, Willard," 277–78; Gielow, *Old Dad Chiro,* 101, 115; Melvin J. Rosenthal, "The Structural Approach to Chiropractic: From Willard Carver to Present Practice," *Chiropractic History,* 1 (1981): 25–26; Rhodes, *Chiropractic in Texas,* 5–6. Charles Ray Parker was the valedictorian of the Palmer class of 1905.

20. Rosenthal, "Structural Approach to Chiropractic," 25–26; see also Dye, *Evolution of Chiropractic,* 21.

21. The text of the letter is printed in Rhodes, *Chiropractic in Texas,* 8–10.

22. Palmer, *Science, Art and Philosophy of Chiropractic,* 75. Dr. Story was Thomas Story, a 1901 graduate of the Palmer School, who apparently was practicing in Duluth, Minn., before his derangement. For a fanciful account of the affair, describing Story's possible abduction and strange wanderings on the West Coast before his cure from Palmer, see Maynard, *Healing Hands,* 28–33.

23. Willard Carver, "Applied Psychology: Lecture No. I, June 11, 1913; Lecture No. II, June 12, 1913; Lecture No. VIII, June 20, 1913," in *Carver's Analysis of Relatolity: As Applied to Psychology, Biology, and Physiology,* 3 vols. (Oklahoma City: by the author, 521 West Ninth Street, North, 1940), 1:4–8, 10–11, 14–19, 39, 199–200.

24. Carver, "Applied Psychology: Lecture No. IV, n.d.; Lecture No. VIII, June 20, 1913," in *Carver's Analysis of Relatolity,* 1:62–63, 76–77, 187–89, 193–202. In his diary, Carver described an experience of "independent telepathy": on August 28, 1895, when miles away from his sick wife in a hotel room, he saw visions of her and through the night suffered intense pain, which subsided at 7:30 A.M. Returning home, he found that she had died at precisely 7:30. It seems reasonable to assume that this experience led him to examine telepathy and provided him with personal confirmation of telepathic reality.

One source (Rhodes, *Chiropractic in Texas,* 10) claimed that Carver had planned on bringing out Relatolity as early as 1894 but gave no source for the assertion. A Carver diary entry (p. 14) indicated his acceptance of the chiropractic "discovery" in September 1895 and mentioned nothing about Relatolity. The Carver "personal diary" (name given to the material by Logan Archives), however, is actually a collection of reminiscences and not a diary per se.

25. Lee Papers, Misc. Manuscripts, Palmer College Archives. In *Science, Art and Philosophy of Chiropractic,* 233, D.D. Palmer explicitly rejected any notion that chiropractic is only a branch of the healing art or of medicine.

26. Langworthy gave Palmer the normal $500 enrollment tuition in July 1901, probably convinced of the value of chiropractic after Palmer reputedly cured his wife of insanity through two weeks of adjustments earlier in the year for a

charge of $15. Palmer claimed that he was the first to discover that displaced vertebrae caused insanity. See "Chiropractic Rays of Light," *The Chiropractor* 1 (June 1905), reprinted in B.J. Palmer, *History Repeats,* 20; cf. Merwyn V. Zarbuck, "A Profession for 'Bohemian Chiropractic': Oakley Smith and the Evolution of Naprapathy," *Chiropractic History* 6 (1986): 79.

27. Russell W. Gibbons, "Solon Massey Langworthy: Keeper of the Flame during the 'Lost Years' of Chiropractic," *Chiropractic History* 1 (1981): 15–19; *Who's Who in Chiropractic,* 2d ed., s.v. "Langworthy, Solon M.," p. 274; [Thomas], "Topical Index of Lerner's Reports," entry for vol. 5, pp. 334–51. Oakley Smith's *Naprapathic Genetics* (1932) is actually a reissue of the 1906 edition of *Modernized Chiropractic* except for a new, sixteen-page prologue. Smith claimed that the term *modernized chiropractic* was actually a misnomer, a reaction against Palmer chiropractic and the first stage pointing to *his* truly scientific innovation of Naprapathy, the "discovery" that tight ligaments cause disease.

28. Gibbons, "Solon Massey Langworthy," 19–20; [Thomas], "Topical Index of Lerner's Reports," entry for vol. 5, pp. 334–51, 355, 392, Lee Papers, Palmer College Archives. On the Amplia-thrill, see Smith, *Naprapathic Genetics* [*Modernized Chiropractic*], 2:174–79. The word *thrill* in this context means rapid, intermittent traction.

D.D. Palmer (*Science, Art and Philosophy of Chiropractic,* 146) denounced a host of appliances promoted by "A Chiropractic college," probably the American School, and derided the devices as a chiropractic "mixup," spawned from their "paternal sire, Old Allopathy." Antagonism between the Langworthy school and the Palmers included charges that Langworthy and his duplicitous colleagues had plagiarized or stolen a testimonial letter from a grateful patient to D.D. Palmer and inserted Langworthy's name in place of Palmer's. See comments by Rev. Samuel H. Weed, "Memorial Service: In Respect to Dr. D.D. Palmer, Discoverer of Chiropractic, October 23, 1913, at the P.S.C.," *The Chiropractor* 9 (December 1913), reprinted in B.J. Palmer, *History Repeats,* 156.

29. "Autobiography of Oakley Smith," Chicago College of Naprapathy, 1966 (typescript), quoted in "Oakley's Smith's Five Lost Years in Chiropractic, *Chiropractic History* 6 (1986): 23; Smith, *Naprapathic Genetics* [*Modernized Chiropractic*], 1:7–9; *Who's Who in Chiropractic,* 2d ed., s.v. "Smith, Oakley G.," pp. 273–74; Zarbuck, "Oakley Smith and the Evolution of Naprapathy," 77–81. According to Smith (*Naprapathic Genetics,* 10), the word *Naprapathy* meant "to correct disease," from "napra" meaning "to correct" and *pathy* meaning "disease." Smith had attended the University of Iowa medical school sporadically from 1901 to 1903, concentrating on anatomy and physiology, which gave him some background for his work.

Readers of Zarbuck's article should be wary. Zarbuck listed Smith's death as 1955, twelve years premature; cited conflicting dates for Smith's discovery; and concluded that Smith went to Chicago in 1905, a highly unlikely conclusion based on scanty, circumstantial evidence. The editor's photographic montage on p. 76, facing the beginning of the article, includes actual illustrations and quotations from two of Smith's own works, which are more reliable for determining the facts.

For D.D. Palmer's blast at Naprapathy, see *Science, Art and Philosophy of Chiropractic,* 780, 884–85. Palmer seemed less concerned with defections that reputedly established new cures with new names than he was with departures that retained a chiropractic association because the latter practiced an adulterated version that confused the public and watered-down "true" chiropractic.

30. Palmer, *Science, Art and Philosophy of Chiropractic,* 233, 286; quotes from *Neuropathy* are taken from Palmer, p. 147. For a description of medical influence in early chiropractic, see Russell W. Gibbons, "Physician-Chiropractors: Medical Presence in the Evolution of Chiropractic," *Bulletin of the History of Medicine* 55 (Summer 1981): 233–45.

31. R.P. Beideman, "Seeking the Rational Alternative: The National College of Chiropractic from 1906 to 1982," *Chiropractic History* 3 (1983): 17–18; D. Patrick Montgomery and J. Marlene Nelson, "Evolution of Chiropractic Theories of Practice and Spinal Adjustment, 1900–1950," *Chiropractic History* 5 (1985): 74. For a photo of the dissection amphitheatre at the National School, see "Miscellany," *Chiropractic History* 4 (1984): 23.

32. In a memorial article on his life *Medical Octopus* is described as a term used frequently by B.J. *Chiropractic Health Bulletin,* no. 117 (June 1961), The Haldeman Chiropractic Clinic, Pretoria, Logan College of Chiropractic Archives, Chesterfield, Mo.

33. Quoted in Walter I. Wardwell, "The Cutting Edge of Chiropractic Recognition: Prosecution and Legislation in Massachusetts," *Chiropractic History* 2 (1982): 57.

34. A facsimile of the advertisement appeared on the cover of *The North Carolina Chiropractic Journal* 56 (November 1985). An accompanying article, Kathleen A. Crisp, "Chiropractic Lyceums: The Colorful Origins of Chiropractic Continuing Education," 2–7, had first appeared in *Chiropractic History* 4 (1984): 17–22. The parade incident in 1913 which led to the car incident seems to be the forerunner to the lyceum series started in 1914.

35. B.J. mentioned the attendance figure in his lecture before the third annual lyceum in 1916, reprinted in *History Repeats,* 722. The various speakers are mentioned in Dye, *Evolution of Chiropractic,* 301, and Turner, *Rise of Chiropractic,* 43–44.

36. David D. Palmer, *The Palmers* (Davenport, Iowa: Bawden Bros., 1977), 175.

37. A photographic reproduction of the ad appeared in Crisp, "Chiropractic Lyceums," *North Carolina Chiropractic Journal,* 4, and in Crisp, *Chiropractic History,* 16.

38. Gibbons, "Rise of the Chiropractic Educational Establishment," 346. For discussion of Reagan's stint at WOC, see Garry Wills, *Reagan's America: Innocents at Home* (Garden City, NY: Doubleday & Co., 1987), 99–100.

39. B.J. Palmer, *History Repeats,* 230. *Who's Who in Chiropractic,* 2d ed., s.v. "Evins, Dossa D.," p. 313. In 1960, investigators at the Stanford Research Institute found that readings on the dial of the Neurocalometer could be changed dramatically by applying varying degrees of pressure as the device passed down the spine. See Ralph Lee Smith, "Chiropractic: Science or Swindle?" *Today's Health* (May 1965): 56. Smith is viciously antichiropractic; his *judgments* should be considered cautiously.

40. Turner, *Rise of Chiropractic,* 40; Morris Fishbein, "Chiropractic," *Ameri-*

can Mercury (May 1925): 28. On Abrams and the Oscilloclast, see James Harvey Young, *The Medical Messiahs: A Social History of Health Quackery in Twentieth-Century America* (Princeton: Princeton University Press, 1967): 137–42.

41. "More About Neurocalometer Service: Twice a Year Inspection," *Fountain Head News* (August 2, 1924), reprinted in B.J. Palmer, *History Repeats*, 242; Turner, *Rise of Chiropractic*, 39–45; Dye, *Evolution of Chiropractic*, 209–12. There is a discrepancy among the sources over the price of the NCM. By October 1924, New York chiropractors noted the price as $2,000. See letter of New York Chiropractic Association President Lyndon E. Lee to association members, October 8, 1924, and George M. Devinny to Lyndon E. Lee, October 15, 1924, Lee Papers, 1924 Correspondence, Palmer College Archives. B.J. offered the device initially for $620 and periodically raised the price as a way of nudging potential subscribers to lease before another price hike. On December 15, 1924, B.J. wrote to a prospective student: "The neurocalometer is not sold, but is leased for a period of ten years. As you may know, the original lease price for ten years was $620, soon increased to $1,200, later to $1,500, and then to the present price of $2,200, with the prospect of an increase at an early date to $3,000." Quoted in Fishbein, "Chiropractic," 28–29.

42. B.J. Palmer, *History Repeats*, 241–42, 256, 258, 266ff.

43. Although an actual text of the speech itself has failed to surface, the basic content can be reconstructed from various sources. See "Dropping by the Wayside—and Why," *Fountain Head News* (October 24, 1925), reprinted in B.J. Palmer, *History Repeats*, 367ff; Willard J. Danforth to Z.L. Wilcox, September 8, 1924, George M. Devinny to Lyndon E. Lee, October 15, 1924, and Lee to "Dear Doctor," October 20, 1924, Lee Papers, 1924 Correspondence, Palmer College Archives; B.J. Palmer to M.L. Garfunkel, April 29, 1941, quoted in Crisp, "Chiropractic Lyceums," *North Carolina Chiropractic Journal*, 5. Crisp stated incorrectly (p. 4) that B.J. "introduced" the NCM at the 1924 lyceum. The 1924 lyceum actually intensified the prior controversy.

44. "Resolution," n.d. (probably September or October 1924), Board of Directors of the New York State Branch of the Universal Chiropractors Association, Lee Papers, 1924 Correspondence, Palmer College Archives. B.J. was incensed that this resolution got out.

45. Quoted in Fishbein, "Chiropractic," 29.

46. Lyndon E. Lee to "Dear Doctor," October 8, 1924, and Lee to G.W. Rice [Fall 1924], Lee Papers, 1924 Correspondence, Palmer College Archives.

47. Chester C. Stowell, "Lincoln College and the 'Big Four': A Chiropractic Protest, 1926–1962," *Chiropractic History* 3 (1983): 75–78; Dye, *Evolution of Chiropractic*, 137–38. The "Big Four" are mentioned in a letter questioning B.J.'s leadership from H.A. Call to B.J. Palmer, October 8, 1934, Lee Papers, Public Relations Materials, Palmer College Archives.

Dye noted (pp. 138–40) that, for a time, Lincoln College sponsored the Abrams Oscilloclast, offering it as an alternative to B.J.'s Neurocalometer.

48. [B.J. Palmer], *Fountain Head News* 21 (October 1934): 1; Earl C. Bailey to B.J. Palmer, October 9, 1934, Lee Papers, Public Relations Material, Palmer College Archives.

49. *Fountain Head News* 15 (June 18, 1927): 1, quoted in Crisp, "Chiroprac-

tic Lyceums," *North Carolina Chiropractic Journal*, 5. B.J. also sought to consolidate his support through "Neurocalometer Clubs." See *History Repeats*, 270–71.

50. Aristotle, *The Nicomachean Ethics*, quoted in Peter M. Blau, "Exchange Theory," in *The Sociology of Organizations: Basic Studies*, eds. Oscar Grusky and George A. Miller (New York: Free Press, 1970), 133.

51. Dye, *Evolution of Chiropractic*, 212–13; cf. Chrisp, "Chiropractic Lyceums," *North Carolina Chiropractic Journal*, 5–6. Somewhat in sport, *Time* magazine (March 18, 1940, p. 55) mentioned these last three devices in "Cosmic Chiropractor," a piece noting the 95th anniversary of D.D. Palmer's birth.

52. Palmer, *Science, Art and Philosophy of Chiropractic*, 490.

53. E. Ruscheweyh and E.A. Ernest, comps., *Chromaray: The Scientific Way to Health with the* SEVEN COLORS *of the* SPECTRUM (Milwaukee: Ernest Distributing Co., 1937), preface, pp. 2–6, 12–22, Logan College of Chiropractic Archives, Chesterfield, Mo.

54. *Polysine Philosophy: The Story of the McIntosh Polysine Generator and its Place in Physical Therapy Practice* (Chicago: McIntosh Electrical Corp., 1929), 5–69 passim, Logan College Archives.

55. These devices are displayed in the archives of Logan College.

56. F.C. Ellis, *Micro-Dynamics*, 4th ed. (Chicago: Ellis Research Laboratories, 1935), 66–70.

57. "Machinery is good," Emerson wrote in his journal, "but mother wit is better. Telegraph, steam, and balloon and newspaper are like spectacles on the nose of age, but we will give them all gladly to have back again our young eyes." Quoted in John F. Kasson, *Civilizing the Machine: Technology and Republican Values in America, 1776–1900* (New York: Penguin Books, 1977), 131.

58. Young, *Medical Messiahs*, 258–59; R.L. Smith, "The Hucksters of Pain," *The Saturday Evening Post* (August 24, 1963): 86–87.

59. For divisions within the regulars, Thomsonians, and homeopaths, see William G. Rothstein, *American Physicians in the Nineteenth Century: From Sects to Science* (Baltimore: Johns Hopkins University Press, 1972), 61–62, 142–46, 239–43; on homeopaths, see also Martin Kaufman, *Homeopathy in America: The Rise and Fall of a Medical Heresy* (Baltimore: Johns Hopkins University Press, 1971), 116–22, 175; on osteopaths, see Norman Gevitz, *The D.O.'s: Osteopathic Medicine in America* (Baltimore: Johns Hopkins University Press, 1982), 61–74.

60. Paul Starr, *The Social Transformation of American Medicine* (New York: Basic Books, 1982), 92.

CHAPTER FOUR. THE CHILL OF THE LAW

1. "Rain Stops Jail Serenade: Imprisoned Chiropractor's Friends Bring Chicken Instead," *New York World*, May 12, 1924. The Hudson County Chiropractic Society planned a parade upon his release. See "Chiros to Celebrate Release Of Conover," *New York City Journal*, June 5, 1924.

2. Dye, *Evolution of Chiropractic*, 87, 94. Chittenden Turner, *Rise of Chiropractic*, 289–90, noted that, of approximately fifteen thousand cases against chiropractors in the United States to 1924, less than one-fifth were judged guilty.

The enforcement of medical licensure laws was problematic long before chiropractic was invented. Unlicensed practitioners who commanded any local popularity frequently went free. See Samuel L. Baker, "Physician Licensure Laws in the United States, 1865–1915," *Journal of the History of Medicine and Allied Sciences* 39 (April 1984): 183–84.

3. Walter R. Rhodes, *The Official History of Chiropractic in Texas* (Austin: Texas Chiropractic Association, 1978), 74, 77–80.

4. Ibid., 46, 52, 49; *Who's Who in Chiropractic*, 2d ed., s.v. "Lemly, Charles C.," 294, and "Drain, James R.," 286–87.

5. "Chiropractors Open Fight for Licenses," *New York Journal and American*, February 16, 1939. "Chiropractor Declared Law Breaker," in the *New York City Journal* of June 12, 1924, reported that "prominent residents" of Freeport testified to cures resulting from adjustments by Carl P. Nelson. Still, Nelson was convicted of medical practice without a state license, the first conviction of its kind in Nassau County. For the typical defense and for specific ailments patients claimed their chiropractors cured, see Rhodes, *Chiropractic in Texas*, 41, 66–68.

6. This assessment of the American Bureau of Chiropractic is Turner's in *Rise of Chiropractic*, 174. Turner gave the platform on pp. 173–74; generally see pp. 172–77 on the ABC. See also Dye, *Evolution of Chiropractic*, 99–100; *Who's Who in Chiropractic*, 2d ed., s.v. "Werner, William H.," 307; David D. Palmer, *The Palmers* (Davenport, Iowa: Bawden Bros., 1977), 100. Turner had the ABC beginning in 1925, but the generally reliable *Who's Who* placed it in 1927, as did Harold W. Evans, *Historical Chiropractic Data* (n.p., [1979]), 24. David Palmer put the ABC's beginning only "during the years following WWI."

7. Rhodes, *Chiropractic in Texas*, 66–68.

8. Martha M. Metz, *Fifty Years of Chiropractic Recognized in Kansas* (Abilene, Kans.: Shadinger-Wilson, 1965), 25–26. The book is written in a folksy style and, although the testimony and Morris's closing remarks are enclosed in quotation marks, the comments are not taken from a verbatim transcription of the trial but apparently represent the recollection of a courtroom witness. Metz also failed to give the date of the trial, but the context indicates that it occurred sometime in 1911.

The arrest of female chiropractors was not uncommon. Gladys Ingram, a 1915 Palmer graduate who practiced in Cherokee, Iowa, for five years and then in Trenton, Missouri, was arrested twice for practicing medicine, cases both dismissed for "lack of convicting evidence." See the typescript, biographical sketch of Ingram by Marjorie Allen in the Ingram Papers, Palmer College Archives. Mrs. Julia Ruccione of Brooklyn was convicted for illegally practicing medicine and chose to pay a $500 fine rather than spend thirty days in jail. See "Chiropractor Pays $500 Fine In Court," *Brooklyn Eagle*, May 29, 1924.

9. Turner, *Rise of Chiropractic*, 125–26.

10. For the idea of trial publicity as free advertising, see Rhodes, *Chiropractic in Texas*, 70.

11. Quoted in Rothstein, *American Physicians in the Nineteenth Century*, 144.

12. Kaufman, *Homeopathy in America*, 91.

13. Rhodes, *Chiropractic in Texas*, 47–48. Rhodes mentioned the lack of shame and chiropractors who gave adjustments in jail on p. 44.

14. For a brief, general discussion of how the radicalizing experience and

"bearing witness" are important to social movements, see Irwin Unger, *The Movement: A History of the American New Left* (New York: Harper & Row, 1974), 44–45.

15. Dye, *Evolution of Chiropractic*, 95. For examples of chiropractic convictions, see "A Severe Sentence," *Brooklyn New York Citizen*, April 15, 1924; "Quacks in Quake As Chiropractor Draws Cell Term," *New York City News*, May 24, 1924; "Miss Brown's Suit Against Dr. Shyne For $50,000 Opens," *Utica New York Dispatch*, May 20, 1924; "Woman Wins $10,000 From Ex-Brooklynite [Shyne] in Chiropractic Suit," *Brooklyn New York Times*, May 26, 1924.

16. "Chiropractic Sunbeams," *The Davenport Democrat and Leader*, n.d., ca. April 8, 1906; a transcription of the majority of the article is given in Gielow, *Old Dad Chiro*, 110–13. There was nothing novel about Palmer's religious analogy. Homeopathic and botanical practitioners had used the same defense in the nineteenth century. See Rothstein, *American Physicians in the Nineteenth Century*, 169 n. 43.

17. 221 Mass. 184, 108 N.E. 893 (1915).

18. The concept of excluding certain practitioners from licensing requirements, especially those who seemed to possess a "cunning" from above, was certainly nothing new. A 1542 British statute exempted certain "honest" domestic practitioners who were considered to be endowed by God with curative knowledge and power. See Joseph F. Kett, *Formation of the American Medical Profession: The Role of Institutions, 1780–1860* (New Haven: Yale University Press, 1968), 4.

19. Commonwealth v. Porn, 196 Mass. 326, 82 N.E. 31 (1907); Commonwealth v. Jewelle, 199 Mass. 558, 85 N.E. 858 (1908).

20. Other state supreme courts followed the reasoning of the Zimmerman case, usually where statutes also defined medical practice in broad terms. For example, see Louisiana Board of Medical Examiners v. Fife, 162 La. 681, 111 So. 58, 54 A.L.R. 594 (1926) at pp. 596 and 597 of the A.L.R. For other rulings that chiropractic constitutes medical practice within the bounds of state law, see Parks v. State, 159 Ind. 211, 64 N.E. 862 (1902); State v. Johnson, 84 Kan. 411, 114 P. 390 (1911); State v. Morrison, 98 W.Va. 289, 127 S.E. 75 (1925); Whipple v. Grandchamp 261 Mass. 40, 158 N.E. 270, 57 A.L.R. 974 (1927).

For the problems of chiropractic in Massachusetts, see Walter I. Wardwell, "The Cutting Edge of Chiropractic Recognition: Prosecution and Legislation in Massachusetts," *Chiropractic History* 2 (1982): 55–65.

21. The ten states were Illinois, Arkansas, Georgia, Idaho, Mississippi, Ohio, Pennsylvania, Rhode Island, North Carolina, and Tennessee. See [B.J. Palmer, ed.], *Here Are The Facts* (n.p., n.p., 1921), 15. B.J. also included New York in the list; in People v. Ellis, 162 App. Div. 288 (1912), however, the court ruled that the appellant chiropractor's actions fell within the statutory definition of medical practice. See *New York State Journal of Medicine* 24 (January 1924): 39.

For particular court cases, see especially State v. Gallagher, 101 Ark. 593, 143 S.W. 98 (1912), and Harris v. State, 229 Miss. 755, 92 So. 2d 217 (1957).

22. Where general words follow a specific enumeration, the general words are to be held to things of the same general kind or class and not construed in their widest extent. See *Black's Law Dictionary*, 5th ed., s.v. "Ejusdem generis." See also 61 Am. Jur. 2d, Physicians, Surgeons, and Other Healers, section 44.

23. A copy of the "Memorandum of Judge Lansden's Opinion" is given in [Palmer, ed.], *Here Are the Facts, 9.*

24. People v. Love, 298 Ill. 304, 131 N.E. 809, 16 A.L.R. 703 (1921).

25. See 61 Am. Jur. 2d, Physicians, Surgeons, and Other Healers, section 13. *Quo warranto* involves a legal proceeding designed to recover an office, franchise, or privilege from an individual who held it previously.

26. Richard Harrison Shryock, *Medical Licensing in America, 1650–1965* (Baltimore: Johns Hopkins University Press, 1967), vii; Richard Harrison Shryock, *Medicine and Society in America, 1660–1860* (New York: New York University Press, 1960), 11.

27. David Freeman Hawke, *Everyday Life in Early America* (New York: Harper & Row, 1988), 85. Shryock, *Medicine and Society in America,* 34–35; Kett, *Formation of the American Medical Profession,* 11. Shryock argued (*Medical Licensing in America,* 8–9) that the training and practice of rural American doctors was similar to that of many of the English village surgeons or apothecaries who tended most Englishmen; that distinctions between medical orders broke down in England as well as in America because "similar environments encouraged similar behavior on both sides of the Atlantic."

28. Quoted in Shryock, *Medical Licensing in America,* 5.

29. Robert C. Derbyshire, *Medical Licensure and Discipline in the United States* (Baltimore: Johns Hopkins University Press, 1969), 3–6; Kett, *Formation of the American Medical Profession,* 12–31; Starr, *Social Transformation of American Medicine,* 56–59; Duffy, *The Healers,* 69, 175–77; Rothstein, *American Physicians in the Nineteenth Century,* 72–80.

30. Shryock, *Medical Licensing in America,* 47.

31. Baker, "Physician Licensure Laws in the United States," 173–97. Baker's work is the most thorough, concise study of the subject for the period 1865–1915. See also Ronald Hamowy, "The Early Development of Medical Licensing Laws in the United States, 1875–1900," *The Journal of Libertarian Studies* 3 (1979): 73–119.

32. Nathan O. Hatch, "Introduction: The Professions in a Democratic Culture," in *The Professions in American History,* ed. Nathan O. Hatch (Notre Dame, Ind.: University of Notre Dame Press, 1988), 1, 2. Don K. Price, "The Profession of Government Service," in ibid., 163–64, also defined the term *profession* in a similar fashion. See also Eliot Friedson, "Are Professions Necessary?" in *The Authority of Experts: Studies in History and Theory,* ed. Thomas L. Haskell (Bloomington: Indiana University Press), 3–27. This viewpoint is the classical, liberal understanding of what constitutes a profession and stands in opposition to a Marxian framework. As Haskell explained in his introduction to *The Authority of Experts* (p. xx), "the liberal tends to identify experts as people who, because they have special knowledge and skills, also acquire power and prestige; while the Marxian tends to identify them as members of classes who, because they are favorably situated in society-wide systems of dominance and submission, also possess valuable knowledge and skills."

33. Bruce Sinclair, "Episodes in the History of the American Engineering Profession," in *The Professions in American History,* ed. Hatch, 129; Michael Schudson, "The Profession of Journalism in the United States," in ibid., 145–46.

34. Laurence Veysey, "Higher Education as a Profession: Changes and Continuities," in ibid., 17–18.

35. Burton J. Bledstein, *The Culture of Professionalism: The Middle Class and the Development of Higher Education in America* (New York: W.W. Norton, 1976), 111, 90, 92, 78–80, 67. See also Harold L. Wilensky, "The Professionalization of Everyone?" *The American Journal of Sociology* 70 (September 1964): 137–58.

36. "Plumbing is no longer merely a trade," Andrew Young explained to the American Public Health Association in an 1891 address. "Its importance and value in relation to health, and its requirements regarding scientific knowledge, have elevated it to a profession." Andrew Young, "The Relations of the Plumbers and the Physicians," *Public Health, Philadelphia* 17 (1891): 48, quoted in Barbara Gutmann Rosenkrantz, "Cart before Horse: Theory, Practice and Professional Image in American Public Health, 1870–1920," *Journal of the History of Medicine and Allied Sciences* 29 (January 1974): 60.

37. William Lutz, *Doublespeak: From "Revenue Enhancement" to "Terminal Living": How Government, Business, Advertisers, and Others Use Language to Deceive You* (New York: Harper & Row, 1989): 20, 109.

38. Quoted in Nathan O. Hatch, "Introduction: The Professions in a Democratic Culture," in *The Professions in American History,* ed. Hatch, 3.

39. Thomas L. Haskell, *The Emergence of Professional Social Science: The American Social Science Association and the Nineteenth-Century Crisis of Authority* (Urbana: University of Illinois Press, 1977), 13, vi, 39, 62.

40. Starr, *Social Transformation of American Medicine,* 102–3.

41. David B. Truman, *The Governmental Process: Political Interests and Public Opinion* (New York: Alfred A. Knopf, 1951), 358.

42. "Report of the Chiropractors' Convention of the East, June 21st and June 22nd, 1924," 19–21 (typescript), in Lee Papers, Misc. Manuscripts: folder #2, Palmer College Archives.

43. Quoted in James G. Burrow, *Organized Medicine in the Progressive Era: The Move toward Monopoly* (Baltimore: Johns Hopkins University Press, 1977), 68.

44. *Buffalo Evening News,* May 12, 1927.

45. Untitled MS, Lee Papers, Misc. Manuscripts: folder #1, Palmer College Archives.

46. Truman, *Governmental Process,* 245. See also pp. 50–51, 214–45 passim.

47. "The Original Copy of B.J. Palmer's Address Before The New York State Chiropractic Society, November 14, 1915," p. 6, in Lee Papers, "Items for Special Presentation to Palmer College," Misc. Material, Palmer College Archives. Dye, *Evolution of Chiropractic,* 227, made the point that B.J. was never a "keen advocate of legislative recognition" for chiropractic because legislation restricted choice. Dye also noted, p. 97, that internal differences over what constituted chiropractic hindered legislation and "that there were many heated discussions, often terminating in blows between the members."

Although he falls into the simple straight/mixer dichotomy, Wardell, "Cutting Edge of Chiropractic Recognition," 60, noted that "the main effect of the split between straights and mixers in Massachusetts as elsewhere, was to make agreement on the kind of licensing law to be proposed nearly impossible to achieve." For a bitter battle over a healing arts statute between B.J. Palmer and "mixer" W.A.

Budden, see Meridel I. Gatterman, "W.A. Budden: The Transition through Proprietary Education, 1924–1954," *Chiropractic History* 2 (1982): 22.

48. The license was issued to Roy Wood of Minot in April 1915. See Metz, *Fifty Years of Chiropractic*, 38; for the politics of passage in Kansas, see pp. 30–42. Legal maneuvering by the governor and state attorney general delayed the appointment of a chiropractic board of examiners in Kansas until May 1915. See also Burrow, *Organized Medicine in the Progressive Era*, 69–70.

49. Rhodes, *Chiropractic in Texas*, 123–24.

Andrew K. Berger, "A Chronology of Chiropractic Licensing in the United States and the District of Columbia," *Research Forum: A Journal of Chiropractic Research* 3 (Spring 1987): 83, wrote that "no geographical trends are apparent from the chronology." However, there is a basic geographical trend that he missed. The licensing pattern indicates a movement from Midwest to West with some strength in the upper South and little in the Northeast, a course that in 1931 Turner (*Rise of Chiropractic*, p. 99) also noticed. Berger mistakenly placed the beginning of licensing in Kansas in 1957, apparently confusing the passage of a basic science law for chiropractors in that year with the beginning of licensing. Table I, p. 79, purports to list the fifty states and the District of Columbia "by the order in which their licensing boards reported they began to license chiropractic." The table, however, is inconsistent. The date legislation passed rather than the beginning of licensing sometimes determines the order. For example, Berger noted that California passed legislation on December 21, 1922, and issued the first license on February 28, 1923 (p. 81) and then entered the date in Table I as December 21, 1922. In Massachusetts, on the other hand, legislation passed on June 28, 1966, and the first license was issued on March 22, 1967 (p. 82), and Berger entered the date in Table I as March 22, 1967. In a two-paragraph discussion concluding the article, Berger described a "slow growth of legalization," and in the next sentence noted that twenty-eight states (his own data in Table I actually indicate thirty, not counting Kansas, which he missed) began licensing from 1915 to 1923, hardly "slow growth." Nevertheless, these points are relatively minor; Berger compiled useful data by surveying the state chiropractic licensing boards.

50. See Stephen Jay Gould, *The Mismeasure of Man* (New York: W.W. Norton, 1981), 192–233. Gould, of course, pointed out the highly dubious nature of these tests and the hereditarian conclusions drawn but noted the tests' influence in directing social policy.

51. *New York State Journal of Medicine* quoted by Lyndon Lee in "Why Drugless Methods," Lee Papers, Misc. Manuscripts: folder #2, Palmer College Archives; "Text of Dr. Lyndon E. Lee's Address To The Graduating Class Of The Standard School of Chiropractic, May 21st, 1925," 3 (typescript), in Lee Papers, Misc. Manuscripts: folder #1.

52. See "B.J. Palmer's Address Before the New York State Chiropractic Society," 10–15, 39–51, in Lee Papers, Misc. Material, Palmer College Archives.

53. Turner, *Rise of Chiropractic*, 96. For discussion of licensing as of 1930, see pp. 95–120.

54. Metz, *Fifty Years of Chiropractic*, 50, 100, 129–30. In the 1957 session, the Kansas legislature also established a Composite Healing Arts Board composed

of eleven members—three chiropractors, three osteopaths, and five medical men—with a quorum set at seven (p. 116).

By 1976, Nebraska still had only eighty-one resident chiropractors; by 1985 the number of licensed chiropractors had increased to only 221. For these figures and for figures in all states for 1976, 1981, and 1984, see "U.S. Distribution of Doctors of Chiropractic," *ICA (International Chiropractic Association Review)* (May–June 1986): 6. For 1985 figures, see Palmer College of Chiropractic, Department of Institutional Analysis, "Analysis of Chiropractic Distribution—September, 1985" (typescript).

55. Albert Q. Maisel, "Can Chiropractic Cure?" *Hygeia* (April 1946): 263.

56. Calculated from figures given in Norman Gevitz, *The D.O.'s: Osteopathic Medicine in America* (Baltimore: Johns Hopkins University Press, 1982), Table 1, p. 86. Gevitz obtained his figures from medical licensure statistics given annually in the *Journal of the American Medical Association;* Gevitz displayed them in three-year increments, 1942–44, 1945–47, 1948–50, and 1951–53. Assuming that the numbers for 1948–50 for chiropractors are listed correctly, Gevitz made a major error in calculating the percentage that passed. He showed 1,489 chiropractic examinees with 224 passing and then calculated the percentage as 35.1. It should be 15.0. In addition, a number of his percentages, although basically accurate, are rounded incorrectly. Gevitz noted that after 1953 results were no longer reported by type of practitioner.

57. Cash Asher, "Medical Straight-Jacket for Chiropractic," *The Nashville News Combined with the Journal of the Tennessee Ass'n of Naturopathic Physicians* 2 (December 1946): 1.

58. In Colorado, chiropractors were licensed by the state medical board from 1915 through 1933, when an independent board of chiropractic examinees issued its first license. Berger, "A Chronology of Chiropractic Licensing," 78, 80.

59. In a popular referendum in 1932, citizens of Massachusetts rejected a proposal to license chiropractors 602,520 to 351,094, or 37.5 percent to 21.8 percent, with 40.7 percent of the ballots blank. Wardwell, "Cutting Edge of Chiropractic Recognition," 62.

60. Lyndon Lee to Delos A. Blodgett, July 24, 1963, Lee Papers, Correspondence, 1955–1976, Palmer College Archives.

CHAPTER FIVE. MISSIONARIES OF HEALTH

1. Mary Deneen, "Loyalty," *The Chiropractor* 6 (December 1910), reprinted in B.J. Palmer, *History Repeats,* 26.

2. Examples of such experiences are legion and remain today an important reason why many become chiropractic students. At the annual convention of the Virginia Chiropractic Association on August 24, 1985, a student from Life Chiropractic College (Marietta, Georgia), formerly a special education teacher in Brooklyn, told me of seeing a "white light" as his first chiropractic adjustment had released him from pain several years earlier. The dramatic deliverance led him to alter his career plans and enroll at Life. Even a casual look at *Who's Who in Chiropractic,* 2d ed., will yield scores of similar testimonials.

In 1960, a Haynes Foundation study by the Stanford Research Institute reported that 42 percent of the chiropractic college students surveyed noted that they became chiropractors because they had benefited personally from chiropractic treatment. See Marcus Bach, *The Chiropractic Story* (Austell, Ga.: Si-Nel Publishing & Sales Co., 1968), 203.

A recent sociological study of chiropractic in Canada (Merrijoy Kelner, Oswald Hall, and Ian Coulter, *Chiropractors: Do They Help?* [Toronto: Fitzhenry & Whiteside, 1980]) reported (p. 44) that "personal contacts with individual chiropractors were highly influential in encouraging [students] to apply to chiropractic college" and (p. 45) that "nearly half of the students in our survey report that they had been treated by chiropractors for health problems before they enrolled in college." For examples in chiropractic literature, see "Recording the 80-Year Legacy of One Family," *Chiropractic History: The Archives and Journal of the Association for the History of Chiropractic* 8 (July 1988): 4; Rhodes, *Chiropractic in Texas,* 103–5, 162–63; Metz, *Fifty Years of Chiropractic,* 25; Ellen M. Gerould, "The History of Logan College of Chiropractic," November 30, 1982, p. 2, Logan College Archives, Chesterfield, Mo. (typescript); A.E. Homewood, "Chiropractic," *University of Toronto Medical Journal* (February 1961); reprint, Ontario Chiropractic Association, n.d., p. 4.

3. Mencken quoted in Marshall Smith, "If Your Back Is Out, You're 'In'," *Life* (April 9, 1965): 77. Both the rate of chiropractic success and dramatic, individual cures sometimes made headlines. The *Clinton* (Iowa) *Daily Advertiser* of May 18, 1911, reported that, "since May 1, 1909, The Palmer School of Chiropractic has enrolled 3,380 patients, many of these being chronic cases who had been given up by all the regular physicians as having but a limited time to live. Out of this number only seven have died, a number which would be only a good average for the same number of people enjoying the best of health." Reprinted in B.J. Palmer, *History Repeats,* 152. Articles clipped from the *St. Louis Daily Globe-Democrat* (June 10, 1942), *The Aurora Beacon-News* (June 28, 1942), and other local newspapers and a testimonial from Ronald's father, all are displayed (along with the actual metal strip taken from the boy's stomach) in the Logan College Archives.

4. "Testimonial Questionnaire" #1156 (February 17, 1955), Logan College Archives.

5. "Hammer Victim Dies," *New York World,* May 12, 1924.

6. Rhodes, *Chiropractic in Texas,* 42.

7. Eric Hoffer, *The True Believer: Thoughts on the Nature of Mass Movements* (New York: Harper & Row, 1951), 21, 20. In contrast to chiropractic, the medical profession (especially the American Medical Association) conforms to what Hoffer calls a "practical organization," which appeals primarily to self-interest.

8. "A Glorious Future," *The Chiropractor* 11 (January 1915), quoted in Russell W. Gibbons, "The Evolution of Chiropractic: Medical and Social Protest in America, Notes on the Survival Years and After," in *Modern Developments in the Principles and Practices of Chiropractic,* ed. Scott Haldeman (New York: Appleton-Century-Crofts, 1980), 12–13. Nutting was Willard Carver's uncle and was very close to B.J. Palmer.

9. "Uncle Howard" Nutting, "U.C.A.—What?" *The Chiropractor* 4 (August–September 1908), reprinted in B.J. Palmer, *History Repeats,* 108.

10. Metz, *Fifty Years of Chiropractic,* 29.

11. Shegetaro Morikubo, "Stray Thoughts on Chiropractic and the P.S.C.," *The Chiropractor* 3 (December–January 1906–7), reprinted in B.J. Palmer, *History Repeats,* 99. B.J. Palmer long exhibited a messianic attitude that attracted a corps of such dedicated disciples who were willing to embrace him without question. His address to the Pre-Lyceum Class on August 19, 1935, carried the plea that had energized converts through the years. "I do not have the physical force to go out and carry my vision and message of Chiropractic into the highways and byways of the world, but I have made it my aim in life to impart this message to the world through you, to teach this message of Chiropractic and its possibilities to you, that you could carry the message and the vision into those highways and byways for me." Verbatim transcription of the address is given in Dye, *Evolution of Chiropractic,* 320.

Chiropractor Arthur Nickson described B.J. as a powerful speaker with "hypnotic eyes" that exerted great influence upon certain people. Interview with Arthur L. and Vi Nickson, Logan College of Chiropractic, Chesterfield, Mo., June 28, 1986.

Staunch lay chiropractic advocate Marcus Bach (*The Chiropractic Story,* 120, 159) characterized his friend B.J. variously as the "dean of chiropractic lore, champion of the chiropractic cause," and as "electric," "contagious," "provocative," and "Supernal."

12. Deneen, "Loyalty," 27; "A Little Chat With the Boys," *The Chiropractor* 5 (March 1909), reprinted in *History Repeats,* 113.

13. Phylis Lan Lin ("The Chiropractor, Chiropractic, and Process: A Study of the Sociology of an Occupation," Ph.D. diss., University of Missouri-Columbia, 1972) studied fifty-eight chiropractors practicing in Missouri and noted (p. 54) that 70.7 percent were Protestant, 17.2 percent were Catholic, 3.4 percent had other religious backgrounds, and 8.7 percent claimed no religious affiliation. Religious affiliation, of course, does not necessarily translate into ardent Christian belief.

Harry Gallaher, *History of Chiropractic: A History of the Philosophy, Art and Science of Chiropractic and Chiropractors in Oklahoma* (Guthrie, Okla.: William E. Welch & William H. Pattie, 1930): 107–76, presented brief, biographical sketches of notable Oklahoma chiropractors. Robert E. Ihne's comment (p. 142) that "a physician or doctor should be first a Christian and then a doctor or physician" probably expressed the view of many. Of 112 entries, 50 include specific religious affiliations: 11 Baptists, 11 Methodists, 8 Christian/Church of Christ members, 8 Presbyterians, 4 Methodist Episcopals, 2 Catholics, 2 Quakers, 1 Lutheran, 1 Nazarene, and 2 from the Reorganized Church of Jesus Christ of Latter-Day Saints. Two others, Arthur L. and Dora Lee Strong, spent two years in Phillips Christian University "preparatory for Evangelistic work." Arthur's ill health halted study, and "he sought relief through Chiropractic and was cured," after which both took up chiropractic (p. 167). Sixty-two of the 112 are not listed with specific religious attachments, which in some cases may simply indicate the compiler's lack of information. These Oklahoma chiropractors, reflecting their profession, were joiners. Many belonged to the Masons, Shriners, and other fraternal bodies.

More recently, *Who's Who in Chiropractic,* 2d ed., specifically requested those featured to list their religion among the biographical information they were asked to supply. Compiling information from the 875 entries (pp. 23–265) produced the following breakdown: No affiliation given (310), 35.4 percent; Catholics (103), 11.8 percent; Protestants (421), 48.1 percent; Jewish (23), 2.6 percent; other religious background, including one self-described "Unitarian Atheist" (18), 2.1 percent.

Metz, *Fifty Years of Chiropractic*, 95, mentioned that a number of chiropractors also served in the ministry and noted that many were Baptists, Methodists, and Church of Christ members. "Most chiropractors," she wrote, "feel they have a special insight on how 'God Will Take Care of You' as the oft-sung song states it." Rhodes, *Chiropractic in Texas*, 83, 86–87, also noted a number of preacher-chiropractors and the strong religious ties within the profession.

The Christian Chiropractors Association was organized in the United States and Canada in the midfifties and, according to the 1986 American Chiropractic Association pamphlet "Chiropractic: State of the Art" (p. 31), "look forward to a constantly enlarging vision of missions." By 1986, the Christian Chiropractors Association was "represented by chiropractic missionaries in Indonesia, Peru, Quebec, Bolivia, Ethiopia, Monaco, Israel, Hong Kong, Mexico, and the United States." The Statement of Faith detailed in the official pamphlet of the Association [n.d., ca. 1988] notes that the group is "conservative in theology," embracing "the cardinal essentials of the historic Christian faith." There is also a Latter-Day Saints Chiropractors Association and at least one "Christian Based Chiropractic Management Seminar," operating from St. Paul, Minnesota, as "RE-NEW-ALL SEMINARS." See advertisement in *The Digest of Chiropractic Economics* (March–April 1986): 72.

14. "Memorial Service: In Respect to Dr. D.D. Palmer, Discoverer of Chiropractic, October 23, 1913, at the P.S.C.," *The Chiropractor* 9 (December 1913), reprinted in B.J. Palmer, *History Repeats*, 158–59. Weed apparently never became a chiropractor himself but stood as a staunch advocate after personal healing under chiropractic care.

15. The primary impetus for antebellum health reform came from a Christianity that turned assaults on immoderation and attendant evils into moral crusades. See James C. Whorton, *Crusaders for Fitness: The History of American Health Reformers* (Princeton: Princeton University Press, 1982), esp. 13–61. Parker's comments are transcribed in "Report of the Chiropractors' Convention of the East, June 21st and June 22nd, 1924," 17–18 (typescript), in Lee Papers, Misc. Manuscripts: folder #2, Palmer College Archives.

16. "A Christian Concept of Chiropractic Philosophy," National Chiropractic Association (NCA) *Journal* (May 1952; rev. and repr. n.p.), in H.L. McSherry Papers, Palmer College Archives. McSherry cited (p. 3) *Footprints of God* by A.I. Brown, which gave the results of a poll on the religious beliefs of the medical profession: 86 percent of the psychologists, 82 percent of the biologists, and 66 percent of the physicists signed themselves as "atheists." Curiously, McSherry did not give the percentage of medical doctors who identified themselves as such.

17. B.J. Palmer, "Paradoxes," lecture delivered before the third annual lyceum, Davenport, Iowa, August 1916, printed in B.J. Palmer, *History Repeats*, 735–37, 741.

18. Dye, *Evolution of Chiropractic*, 183. The July 1943 issue of *Maryland*

Chiropractic News (p. 3) contains an ad for Dr. J. Leslie Jones's "Chiropractic Health Service" in Baltimore. In bold print, the ad proclaims simply, "Colored Patients." It is not clear whether Jones was a black chiropractor offering his services to the black community or whether he was a white chiropractor attempting to cross the chiropractic color line. In either case, the ad underscores the segregated nature of chiropractic.

19. Among 112 chiropractors in Gallaher's biographical gallery (*History of Chiropractic*, 107–76), no black is pictured. In Metz, *Fifty Years of Chiropractic*, the first black chiropractor to be pictured appears on p. 114, a state legislator (1955–57) from Kansas City named Eldred Browne.

20. Bobby Westbrooks, "The Troubled Legacy of Harvey Lillard: The Black Experience in Chiropractic," *Chiropractic History* 2 (1982): 49–51. Westbrooks is founder of the American Black Chiropractic Association.

Blacks who wanted to enter orthodox medicine in the late nineteenth and early twentieth centuries were generally restricted to special medical schools for blacks that began to appear after the Civil War, spurred by the work of the Freedman's Bureau. Many of these schools were short-lived. Before the Flexner Report of 1910, seven such schools existed; after the report, only two survived (Howard in Washington, D.C., and Meharry in Nashville). Scarcity of opportunity (blacks were also usually excluded from internships and hospital privileges) meant that by 1930 only one of every three thousand black Americans was a medical doctor. See Starr, *Social Transformation of American Medicine*, 124; Duffy, *The Healers*, 286.

For the difficulties involved in opening an integrated chiropractic school, see "School for Chiropractors," *Ebony* (December 1946): 17–18. The piece describes the short-lived Reaver School of Chiropractic in Dayton, Ohio (1945–51), founded by Clarence Reaver, a white, 1941 Palmer graduate with an integrated practice. It was Reaver who had pressed B.J. to admit his black patient Dorothy Clark; her rejection prompted Reaver to establish the school. The Montgomery County (Ohio) Chiropractic Association relieved Reaver of his duties as an officer after he opened the school, and rank-and-file chiropractors harassed him constantly.

21. Westbrooks, "Troubled Legacy," 51–52.

22. Virginia A. Wolfenberger, "Comparison of the Participation of Blacks and Females in Chiropractic," *The Digest of Chiropractic Economics* (March–April 1986): 69; Westbrooks, "Troubled Legacy," 52.

23. "The Search for the first 15 'Disciples'," *Chiropractic History* 3 (1983): 23. D.D. Palmer in the *Science, Art and Philosophy of Chiropractic* listed thirteen of the fifteen as the "earliest graduates of Chiropractic" (p. 778) and included a photograph (p. 886) taken at a reunion in December 1902 that pictures D.D. and son B.J. along with five of the pioneer disciples.

On Almeda Haldeman see Scott Haldeman, "Almeda Haldeman, Canada's First Chiropractor: Pioneering the Prairie Provinces, 1907–1917," *Chiropractic History* 3 (1983): 64–67.

The Palmer School supported women's suffrage in the second decade of the century, attested to by huge mottos emblazoned on the administration building chimney: "EQUAL RIGHTS" and "VOTES 4 WOMEN." See photograph in ibid., 58.

24. Metz, *Fifty Years of Chiropractic*, 38–39, 42, 46. Metz gave the gender

breakdown (210 women, 315 men) for 1925 but came up with the erroneous sum of 533. On p. 54, she again mentioned the 533 figure and stated that there were 323 men in that year. Even if the latter citation is accurate, the percentage of women would move downward only 0.6 percent. Metz noted (p. 25) that in 1911 (the first year of its existence) one-third of the members of the Kansas Chiropractic Association were women and (p. 76) that, of the four who served the most terms in the association (to 1965), two were women. Three of the six chiropractic examiners who served the longest terms on the Kansas board were women (p. 59).

A 1922 photograph (in the Logan College Archives) of students at Colvin Chiropractic College in Wichita shows forty-five women among the eighty-seven people pictured.

25. W. John Alloway and Margaret E. Ronkin, "The Social Anthropology of Chiropractic in Washington, D.C.: Project DC/DC," *Chiropractic History* 2 (1982): 12, chart 2.

26. For example, a Palmer School class photo, ca. 1908 (reprinted in *Chiropractic History* 3 (1983): 58), pictures 36 women among 110 graduates. A caption to the picture states erroneously that one-fourth are women, but an actual count shows one-third. In the rotogravure section of the *Des Moines Sunday Capital* for December 5, 1920, was a piece entitled "Chiropractic is not a fad—It is a curative Science," in which a group picture of fifty-four chiropractors includes twenty women. "Brooklynites Graduates of Chiropractic School," *Brooklyn Eagle*, June 21, 1923, noted that fifteen of fifty graduates from the Standard School of Chiropractic in Manhattan were women. A photograph (in the Logan College Archives) of participants at the fourteenth annual convention (June 4–6, 1927) of the Missouri State Chiropractic Association at the Marquette Hotel in St. Louis shows 45 women among 208 chiropractors. The biographical gallery in Gallaher (*History of Chiropractic*, 107–76) includes 37 women among 115 entries.

Women medical school graduates in the first three decades of the century never exceeded 5.4 percent of all medical graduates. See Carol Lopate, *Women in Medicine* (Baltimore: Johns Hopkins University Press, 1968), 193, appendix 1. During the same period, women physicians were never greater than 6 percent of the total. See Mary Roth Walsh, *"Doctors Wanted: No Women Need Apply": Sexual Barriers in the Medical Profession, 1835–1975* (New Haven: Yale University Press, 1977), 186, table 5. Cynthia Fuchs Epstein in *Women's Place: Options and Limits in Professional Careers* (Berkeley and Los Angeles: University of California Press, 1970), 201, table 2, gave the absolute number of women physicians by decade.

27. Comparison is difficult because figures are sketchy and because the fortunes of unorthodox practice fluctuate considerably, creating wide variations from year to year in the number of active practitioners. William G. Rothstein, in *American Physicians in the Nineteenth Century*, 300 n.5, noted that, in 1900, 12 percent of all homeopathic physicians and 17 percent of the students in homeopathic schools were women. Also in 1900, 9 percent of eclectic school students were women.

28. Beard's chief work was *American Nervousness: Its Causes and Consequences* (New York, 1881). For an engaging discussion of Beard's notions, see Haller and Haller, *Physician and Sexuality*, chap. 1. Lewis is quoted in Whorton, *Crusaders for Fitness*, 276.

29. Quoted in Regina Markell Morantz-Sanchez, *Sympathy and Science: Women Physicians in American Medicine* (New York: Oxford University Press, 1985), 5.

30. "Bronx Chiropractor Thinks Her Sex Is Equal of Man in the Profession," *New York Bronx Home News*, June 1, 1924. For speculations on how the attitudes associated with gender and gender itself have affected scientific development, see Evelyn Fox Keller, *Reflections on Gender and Science* (New Haven: Yale University Press, 1985), esp. chap. 4.

31. B.J. Palmer, "Chiropractic Women and What Women Chiropractors Say" (Davenport, Iowa: Palmer School of Chiropractic, 1918), 46, quoted in Theresa Gromala, "Women in Chiropractic: Exploring a Tradition of Equity in Healing," *Chiropractic History* 3 (1983): 60.

The National College of Chiropractic in Chicago offered the regular or "collegiate" course of eighteen months for $650 (with a $50 discount for cash up front) but charged a husband and wife who registered together only $900. Other schools also offered various discounts for family members. See Louis S. Reed, *The Healing Cults: A Study of Sectarian Medical Practice: Its Extent, Causes, and Control* (Chicago: University of Chicago Press, 1932): 43–45. Metz, *Fifty Years of Chiropractic*, 46, noted "the wisdom of the early schools" in providing special rates for married couples.

32. Interview with Arthur L. and Vi Nickson, Logan College, June 28, 1986. Of thirty-seven women pictured in the biographical gallery in Gallaher, *History of Chiropractic*, 107–76, nine are part of husband-wife teams. The names listed for the May 1922 commencement class of New York's Standard School of Chiropractic indicate that four married couples graduated among forty-six total graduates. See Standard School of Chiropractic Commencement Announcement, Wednesday, May 3, 1922, in Lee Papers, Misc. Manuscripts, Palmer College Archives. Rhodes, *Chiropractic in Texas*, 152, noted two husband and wife teams as prominent members of the Old Texas Chiropractic Research Society.

33. Metz, *Fifty Years of Chiropractic*, 104.

34. "History," MS in Logan College Archives, n.d., ca. 1967. In the chiropractic course, the Logan Class of 1940 had only one woman among twelve men. See photograph of class, Logan College Archives.

35. The National Chiropractic Association, *A Brief in Support of a Proposal to Include Chiropractic as an Occupation Essential to the Conduct of the War, and Necessary to the Maintenance of the Health of the Civilian Population, To the War Manpower Commission, Washington, D.C.,* March 1943; W.T. Brown to H.A. Von Neida, July 8, 1943, Lee Papers, Correspondence, 1943–54.

36. Figures for Logan were obtained by counting the number of men and women pictured in class photos housed in the Logan College Archives and for later years in *The Keystone*, the college yearbook. Photos for a few years were not available. Because of staggered enrollments, more than one graduation occurred in some years.

Other scattered evidence from the postwar era reinforces the idea of a vanishing female presence. A 1955 photograph of chiropractic interns and residents at the Spears Chiropractic Hospital in Denver shows only three women among forty-one pictured. *Chiropractic History* 3 (1983): 50. In 1956, the Texas Chiropractic Association established a "Young Chiropractor of the Year Award" for chiropractors under age forty. From 1956 to 1977 inclusive, no woman received the award. Instead, the Ladies Auxiliary played a major role in these years. Rhodes, *Chiropractic in Texas,* 169–70. Names listed in the "Official Directory of the National Chiropractic Association" for 1961 (listed in the NCA *Journal* 31 [September 1961]: 6) indicate that, of forty-eight state delegates to its National House, only two (from Maryland and Missouri) were women. A 1963 survey by the American Chiropractic Association showed that approximately 7 percent of chiropractic students were women. Lan Lin, "The Chiropractor, Chiropractic, and Process," 54 n.4. Metz, *Fifty Years of Chiropractic,* 46, wrote that "the part played by the women chiropractors in the early years of the profession should be an inspiration for the present time [1965]" and lamented that, instead of serving beside her husband as in times past, "more often, the wife might be getting training as a receptionist, to care for the office details that often," she added bravely, "are equally important to the success of the team."

37. "What You Should Know about Chiropractic" (American Chiropractic Association, n.d., c. 1982), 8; "Profile: Mary Jo Marraffa, D.C. Introduces the International Network of Women Chiropractors," *The American Chiropractor* (July 1986): 52, 54; Gromala, "Women in Chiropractic," 59; Wolfenberger, "Blacks and Females in Chiropractic," 71. At Logan, the enrollment in July 1986 stood at 607, 130 women and 477 men.

38. Quoted in Gielow, *Old Dad Chiro,* 120. In the same address, Palmer claimed that nearly three thousand people had a knowledge of chiropractic and were practicing actively. Gielow accepted the figure uncritically, but it is almost certainly inflated. Discounting it considerably, however, still indicates that many early-day chiropractors learned from a preceptor, since the few fledgling schools that existed by 1908 were turning out only a handful of graduates.

39. Nugent quoted in Albert Q. Maisel, "Can Chiropractic Cure?" *Hygeia* (April 1946): 263; B.J. Palmer, *The Chiropractor* (Davenport, Iowa: Palmer School of Chiropractic, 1916): 4–5, quoted in Alana Ferguson and Glenda Wiese, "How Many Chiropractic Schools? An Analysis of Institutions That Offered the D.C. Degree," *Chiropractic History* 8 (July 1988): 28. B.J.'s quote on manufacturing chiropractors is given in Morris Fishbein, *Fads and Quackery in Healing* (Chicago: n.p., 1932): 108.

40. Facsimile of advertisement in *Chiropractic History* 3 (1983): 24.

41. George Creel, "Making Doctors While You Wait," *Harper's Weekly* (April 3, 1915): 319–21. For charges against other apparent diploma mills, see "5 Schools Named as 'Diploma Mills': Delaware Institutions, Operating from New York, Under Suspicion in Pennsylvania," *New York City Telegram,* December 10, 1923; "Diploma Mills Said To Be Here," *New York City Mail,* December 10, 1923; "Spiegel Planned $60 Diplomas, Lawyer Swears," *New York City Tribune,* December 14, 1923.

42. Facsimile of advertisement in *Today's Chiropractic* (July–August 1985): 32. That the ad appeared in *Cosmopolitan* indicates the appeal chiropractic made to women; by 1912, according to Frank Luther Mott in *A History of American Magazines, 1885–1905* (Cambridge: Harvard University Press, 1957): 496, *Cosmo-*

politan had dropped its former muckraking, begun relying heavily on fiction, and started catering to women.

Creel also blasted the National School for its correspondence course but noted that completion resulted in the "Degree of Diplomat" ("whatever that means," he added) rather than the Doctor of Chiropractic degree, which required a three-month resident course. The distinctions were blurry because the "Diplomat" was apparently entitled to treat patients as any chiropractor would. See George Creel, "Easy Money Doctors," *Harper's Weekly* (April 24, 1915): 395, 398.

In 1913, an outcast D.D. Palmer himself approached prospective students on a downtown street corner in Oklahoma City and offered twenty written lectures and a diploma for fifty dollars. See Rhodes, *Chiropractic in Texas*, 32.

43. "The Menace of Chiropractic: Practically no Educational Qualifications Necessary for Matriculation in Chiropractic Colleges," *Journal of the American Medical Association* 80 (March 10, 1923): 715–16. See also Matthew J. Brennan, "Perspectives on Chiropractic Education in Medical Literature," *Chiropractic History* 3 (1983): 25–30. For more recent letters of this nature, see Ralph Lee Smith, *At Your Own Risk: The Case against Chiropractic* (New York: Trident Press, 1969), 69–71.

Eric Hoffer (*True Believer*, 29) noted a "tendency to judge a race, a nation or any distinct group by its least worthy members. Though manifestly unfair, this tendency has some justification. For the character and destiny of a group are often determined by its inferior elements."

For a recent appraisal of the Flexner Report, see Gert H. Brieger, "The Flexner Report: Revised or Revisited?" *Medical Heritage* 1 (January–February 1985): 25–34.

44. Lyndon E. Lee, "The Chiropractic Backbone," *Harper's Weekly* (September 18, 1915): 285–88.

45. Rothstein, *American Physicians in the Nineteenth Century*, 289, 292; Starr, *Social Transformation of American Medicine*, 42–44; Duffy, *The Healers*, 170–75. Duffy mentioned the eight-year-old applicant on p. 261.

46. Starr, *Social Transformation of American Medicine*, 82.

47. E. Richard Brown, "He Who Pays the Piper: Foundations, the Medical Profession, and Medical Education," in *Health Care in America: Essays in Social History*, eds. Susan Reverby and David Rosner (Philadelphia: Temple University Press, 1979), 151; Duffy, *The Healers*, 264.

48. G.W. Hardie to Theodore W. Price, July 23, 1923, reprinted in B.J. Palmer, *History Repeats*, 204–6.

49. Universal Chiropractors' Association Directory [1925], cited by Gari-Anne Patzwald, "Discovering and Recording Chiropractic History: For a Systematic Program in the Profession," *Chiropractic History* 1 (1981): 9 n.9. Ferguson and Wiese, "How Many Chiropractic Schools?" 29, relying on Reed (*Healing Cults*, 36), cited eighty-two schools for 1925, but the UCA Directory is probably more accurate.

50. Russell W. Gibbons, "Chiropractic's Abraham Flexner: The Lonely Journey of John J. Nugent, 1935–1963," *Chiropractic History* 5 (1985): 45–51; *Who's Who in Chiropractic*, 2d ed., s.v. "Nugent, John J.," pp. 313–14.

51. Gibbons, "Chiropractic's Abraham Flexner," 46–48; Ernest G. Napolitano, "The Struggle for Accreditation in Chiropractic: A Unique History of Educational Bootstrapping," *Chiropractic History* 1 (1981): 23–24; "The President's Page," *The Hawkeye Chiropractor* (June 1943), reprinted in *Maryland Chiropractic News* (July 1943), 3. In this piece, H.D. Scanlon, president of the Iowa Chiropractors' Association, sought to correct false statements B.J. had made in an article appearing in the *Fountain Head News* entitled "Bluff and Hooey." At the Iowa state convention B.J. had spoken against higher educational standards, whereas Nugent had spoken for them. B.J. claimed to have crossed swords with Nugent face to face and won the encounter. Scanlon claimed that B.J. was not even in the hall during Nugent's lecture and distorted what happened in his characteristically "egotistical way."

The medical profession was unimpressed with Nugent's code. Joseph D. Wassersug, in "The Case against Chiropractic," *The American Mercury* (February 1950): 165, wrote that Nugent's educational code "reads like a joke-book when it is compared with the standards of regular colleges and medical schools."

52. David D. Palmer, *The Palmers* (Davenport, Iowa: Bawden Bros., 1977), 28, 54.

53. Napolitano, "Struggle for Accreditation," 24; "What You Should Know about Chiropractic," 8–10; Gibbons, "Rise of the Chiropractic Educational Establishment," 349–50. Gibbons attempted a periodization of chiropractic education into four eras: (1) the tutorial period (1897–1905), (2) the classical period (1905–24), (3) the proprietary period (1924–60), and (4) the professional period (1960–   ). The yearly breakdown is probably about as good as any, but both the second and third periods seem misnamed. "Classical" implies the development of a traditional or standardized course, which certainly fails to describe Gibbons's second era. The "proprietary" label is problematic because chiropractic education throughout the two earlier periods was also proprietary.

See also Gibbons, "Chiropractic's Abraham Flexner," 49–50; "Chiropractic: State of the Art" (Arlington, Va.: American Chiropractic Association, 1986), 34–42; R.C. Schafer, *Opportunities in Chiropractic Health Care Careers* (Lincolnwood, Ill.: VGM Career Horizons, 1985), 69–103.

CHAPTER SIX. BONES OF CONTENTION: VERTEBRAE, MONEY, AND AUTHORITY

1. Quoted in Rothstein, *American Physicians in the Nineteenth Century*, 67.
2. See Starr, *Social Transformation of American Medicine*, 3–29 passim.
3. Appendix B contains a listing of chiropractic (popular press) articles in chronological sequence and an explanation of my rating system. In *The Social Transformation of American Medicine* (p. 260), Starr described the 1920s as the decade of heightened agitation against "quackery."
4. For discussion of the postwar increase, see James Playsted Wood, *Magazines in the United States*, 2d ed. (New York: Ronald Press Co., 1956), 325–26.
5. "The Case for Chiropractic," *American Mercury* (February 1950): 150.
6. For discussion of therapeutic dissent in recent holistic health movements, see Starr, *Social Transformation of American Medicine*, 392–93.

The circulation history of *Prevention* magazine, started in 1950 by Jerome Irving Rodale, the premier ideologist of the organic foods movement, provides a barometer of the popularity of alternative health ideas. After sluggish growth in the fifties and early sixties, circulation topped one million in 1971 and by the mideighties ballooned to almost three million. See Whorton, *Crusaders for Fitness*, 332–36.

7. "The Disappearance of Doctors From Small Towns: Irregulars in Small Towns," *JAMA* 88 (February 12, 1927): 505–6. Pusey sent questionnaires to physicians in 283 "average rural counties" selected for him by the secretaries of the state medical societies. He asked for the number of osteopaths in the county and the number of osteopaths in the county for more than ten years and repeated the same questions for chiropractors and then for "other irregular practitioners." Unfortunately, Pusey did not report the groups separately but clumped the results under the single category "irregular practitioners" (p. 506). Nevertheless, the questions he asked indicated that osteopaths and chiropractors were the two irregular groups of greatest concern. At least by 1932, chiropractic was the largest irregular medical group in the country, with some sixteen thousand practitioners. See Reed, *Healing Cults*, 32–34.

On the trends within the medical profession, see Starr, *Social Transformation of American Medicine*, 76–77, 112–27, 355–59. On the maldistribution and declining number of medical doctors after 1910, see also Shryock, *Medical Licensing in America*, 30, 64, 84, 91.

8. Reed, *Healing Cults*, 34–35, 133, table 3A. Reed implied that his examination of these four states can be extrapolated to give a picture of the nation at large. Even within his study, however, the case of Florida violates his own general rule and the assumption that he has provided an accurate snapshot of national distribution is unwarranted. Yet Morris Fishbein (*Fads and Quackery in Healing*, 113) made just this assumption, a fallacy of composition, when he took Reed's figures and wrote that "it has been argued that chiropractors replace physicians and take care of the shortage that exists in small towns. Actually, the chiropractors tend to concentrate in the cities, 39 per cent of them being in cities over 200,000, as contrasted with 26 per cent of physicians."

Joseph B. Treaster, "Chiropractic Comes of Age," *Family Health* (December 1978): 29. A 1980 government-funded FACTS Study found the following distribution of chiropractors: 40 percent in towns with less than 25,000 people, but 17 percent of these were in towns adjacent to cities with more than 25,000; 20 percent in small cities; and over 33 percent in cities or suburbs of more than 100,000. The trend for new graduates was toward an urban practice. See "FACTS Bulletin— United States," *International Chiropractic Association Review* (May–June 1986): 4. The June 17, 1985, *Moline Dispatch* ("Chiro Ranks to Double by 1995") noted that about half of all chiropractors work in cities of 50,000 or less, "though with growing access to hospitals, that may change."

9. "Chiropractors Say Attack By Doctors Is Compliment," *Bronx Home News*, December 16, 1920. K.C. Robinson made a similar point in "Whole Theory of Chiropractic is Baseless Reports the Medical Society," (typescript), in Lee Papers, Misc. Manuscripts: folder #1, Palmer College Archives.

10. Figures from the committee's report, *Medical Care for the American People*,

are given in Starr, *Social Transformation of American Medicine*, 262. The rest of the medical dollar was spent as follows: 23.4 cents to hospitals, 18.2 cents to medicines, 12.2 cents to dentists, 5.5 cents to nurses, and 3.3 cents to public health. The community studies on chiropractic income are cited in Reed, *Healing Cults*, 36, and the $4,200 figure is his estimate (which seems reasonable) based on the sample. Reed, however, made a multiplication error (16,000 practitioners times $4,200) and cited aggregate income as $63 million instead of $67.2 million. The other figures I calculated from the committee's numbers.

11. "I want to tell you that the medical profession is affected with a terrible case of 'pocketbookitis,' " Philip Troupe, editor of the *New Haven* (Conn.) *Union News* told the Chiropractic Convention of the East in 1924, "and as much as I think of Chiropractic, I don't think the most expert adjusting in the world could ever cure them!" In "Report of the Chiropractors' Convention of the East, June 21st and June 22nd, 1924," 22 (typescript), in Lee Papers, Misc. Manuscripts; folder #2, Palmer College Archives.

The fear among doctors of competition with irregulars seems to have been much greater at the turn of the century before the consolidation of medical authority and the reduction of physician to population ratios. In the early part of the century, "overcrowding" was the dominant argument physicians used to explain the poverty of the medical profession. See Gerald E. Markowitz and David Rosner, "Doctors in Crisis: Medical Education and Medical Reform during the Progressive Era, 1895–1915," in *Health Care in America: Essays in Social History*, eds. Susan Reverby and David Rosner (Philadelphia: Temple University Press, 1979), 185–205.

12. George W. Whiteside. "Legal," *New York State Journal of Medicine* 24 (January 1924): 38–39.

13. B.J. Palmer, *A Hole in One* (Davenport, Iowa: Palmer School of Chiropractic, n.d., c. early 1930s), 2, 29–30. See also David D. Palmer, *The Palmers* (Davenport: Bawden Bros., 1977), 102, *Evolution of Chiropractic*, 331–43. Dye explained (p. 338) that strict adherents of HIO did not attempt manual adjustments of misaligned vertebrae below the upper cervical region because they believed that only misalignments in this area could cause nerve impingement, pressure, or irritation. To Dye, HIO was the breakthrough to true, scientific chiropractic but still reaped "the age-old criticism of the medical profession and allied scientific minds" (p. 339).

By the forties and early fifties, chiropractor Leo Spears rivaled B.J. as the most controversial practitioner. For claims of mastery over cancer and myriad diseases, see "SPEARS Announces Results of Research and Treatment of CANCER," n.d., c. 1952, in Alfred R. Knarr Papers, Palmer College Archives. The December 1953 *Cosmopolitan* ("Chiropractic—Science or Quackery?" p. 87) tagged Spears as "the busiest and most controversial chiropractor in the country today." For venom directed at Spears from a medical viewpoint, see Ralph Lee Smith, *At Your Own Risk: The Case against Chiropractic* (New York: Trident Press, 1969), 87–99. For a brief sketch of Spears's life, see *Who's Who in Chiropractic*, 2d ed., s.v. "Spears, Leo," pp. 311–12.

14. B.J. Palmer, *A Hole in One*, 10.

15. Walter I. Wardwell made a similar point in "Social Factors in the Survival of Chiropractic: A Comparative View," in *Sociological Symposium* (Spring 1978),

ed. James K. Skipper, Jr. (Blacksburg, Va.: Virginia Polytechnic Institute and State University), 7.

16. "Chiropractic: State of the Art" (American Chiropractic Association, 1986), 46.

17. "Chiropractic" (Indianapolis: Burton Shields Co., 1927).

18. John McMillan Mennell, Direct Testimony (typescript) at 2089–95, Wilk et al.: Complaint #76C3777 filed October 12 in U.S. District Court for the Northern District of Illinois, Eastern Division, 1976.

19. Synovia is the transparent, lubricating fluid secreted by the membranes of joint cavities.

20. W.H. Kirkaldy-Willis and J.D. Cassidy, "Spinal Manipulation in the Treatment of Low-Back Pain," *Canadian Family Physician* 31 (March 1985): 536–40. For definition of anatomical terms, see Benjamin F. Miller and Claire Brackman Keane, *Encyclopedia and Dictionary of Medicine and Nursing* (Philadelphia: W.B. Saunders Co., 1972).

21. The myelin is a fatlike substance that forms a sheath around some nerve fibers; these fibers are called myelinated or medullated fibers. Fibers without the myelin sheath are known as unmyelinated.

Although the Gate Theory fails to explain the entire range of pain phenomena, it has largely supplanted both the Specificity Theory and the Pattern Theory. See Paul M. Paris and Ronald D. Stewart, eds., *Pain Management in Emergency Medicine* (Norwalk, Conn.: Appleton & Lange, 1988), 4–6.

22. Edmund S. Crelin, in "A Scientific Test of the Chiropractic Theory," *American Scientist* 61 (September–October 1973): 574–80, conducted an elaborate test employing a drill press, torque wrench, volt-ohm-microampere meter, and assorted gadgets on six vertebral columns from cadavers in an attempt to discredit the old chiropractic idea of nerve pressure. He concluded triumphantly (p. 580) that his experimental study "demonstrates conclusively that the subluxation of a vertebra as defined by chiropractic—the exertion of pressure on a spinal nerve which by interfering with the planned expression of Innate Intelligence produces pathology—does not occur." He was probably right that a vertebra cannot press on a nerve. Yet he was battling a straw man; chiropractors no longer believed it either. The failure to realize that chiropractic has evolved and altered itself through the years is a perennial problem of chiropractic adversaries.

23. Kirkaldy-Willis and Cassidy, "Spinal Manipulation," 536, 538; Dalma Heyn, "Chiropractic's New Twist: Is 'Motion Palpation' the Answer to Back Pain?" *Health* (March 1982): 13–14.

Merrijoy Kelner, Oswald Hall, and Ian Coulter, *Chiropractors: Do They Help?* (Toronto: Fitzhenry & Whiteside, 1980), 77, noted that, although the tension between the theory and practice of any health practice is perhaps inescapable, it has been particularly evident in chiropractic, where the skills of practitioners have far outrun the accompanying body of knowledge.

Through 1980, the *Journal of the American Medical Association* noted eighteen instances where chiropractic manipulation had resulted in stroke and pointed out the dangers of manipulation in certain cases. Such a handful, however, would seem to be a highly commendable record given the millions of manipulations that chiropractors have performed. See Robert G. Miller and Robert Burton, "Stroke following Chiropractic Manipulation of the Spine," *JAMA* 229 (July 8, 1974: 189–90, and Kurt P. Schellhas, Richard E. Latchaw, Lyle R. Wendling, and Lawrence H.A. Gold, "Vertebrobasilar Injuries following Cervical Manipulation," *JAMA* 244 (September 26, 1980): 1450–53. The tone of these two articles toward chiropractic was highly muted in comparison to earlier articles in *JAMA,* such as H. Thomas Ballantine, Jr., "Medicine and Chiropractic," *JAMA* 200 (April 17, 1967): 219–23 (a paper read originally before the Third National Congress on Medical Quackery), and Richard P. Bergen, "Cultist Therapy as Criminal Negligence," *JAMA* 196 (June 27, 1966): 249–50.

24. *Chiropractic in New Zealand: Report of the Commission of Inquiry* (Wellington, New Zealand, 1979; repr. ed., Davenport, Iowa: Palmer College of Chiropractic, n.d.), 42–48. For case histories of chiropractic results with type O disorders, see pp. 164–77.

25. U.S. Department of Health, Education, and Welfare, Public Health Service, National Institutes of Health, and the National Institute of Neurological and Communicative Disorders and Stroke Co-operating, *The Research Status of Spinal Manipulative Therapy: A Workshop held at the National Institutes of Health, February 2–4, 1975,* ed. Murray Goldstein, DHEW publication no. (NIH) 76-998, esp. 3–7. Subluxation was defined at the workshop by Joseph Janse ("History of the Development of Chiropractic Concepts; Chiropractic Terminology," 32) as "the alteration of the normal dynamics, anatomical or physiological relationships of contiguous articular surfaces."

Within the medical profession itself, an almost underground manipulative movement has existed at least since the mid-1960s, when the North American Academy of Manipulative Medicine was founded. A group of physical therapists are also devoted to manipulation—a section on Orthopedic Physical Therapy exists within the American Physical Therapy Association. See Walter I. Wardwell, "Discussion: The Impact of Spinal Manipulative Therapy on the Health Care System," in *Research Status of Spinal Manipulative Therapy,* 54. What physicians and therapists deem *manipulation,* however, is often *mobilization.*

26. *Chiropractic in New Zealand,* xii–xiii, 10–17. Because no chiropractic schools exist in New Zealand and most of the nation's practitioners are educated in the United States (typically at Palmer), the report had special significance for American chiropractors. See pp. 82–83.

27. Ibid., 2–5.

28. Dye, *Evolution of Chiropractic,* 113.

29. Carver's figures were cited uncritically in Rhodes, *Chiropractic in Texas,* 56–57. Rhodes simply accepted them as reflecting "a most amazing, almost miraculous state of affairs."

During World War II, the National Chiropractic Association presented bare statistics compiled by a group called the Chiropractic Bureau of Research and Review that reputedly detailed chiropractic success with seven types of ailments: coccygodynia, lumbago, neuritis, rheumatism, sacroiliac sprain, sciatica, and torticollis. One column reported the number of cases, another reported "Complete Recovery or Decided Improvement," and a third gave the percentage of recovery ranging from a low of 79.9 percent for rheumatism to a high of 96.2 percent for torticollis (contracted cervical muscles known commonly as wryneck). See the

National Chiropractic Association, *A Brief in Support of a Proposal To Include Chiropractic as an Occupation Essential to the Conduct of the War, and Necessary to the Maintenance of the Health of the Civilian Population, To the War Manpower Commission, Washington, D.C.,* March 1943, 3.

30. Kirkaldy-Willis and Cassidy, "Spinal Manipulation," 538. The trials are assessed in D. J. Brunarski, "Clinical Trials of Spinal Manipulation: A Critical Appraisal and Review of the Literature," *Journal of Manipulative and Physiological Therapeutics* 7 (1984): 243–49. The manipulations reported were not all performed by chiropractors, and in most cases the precise technique was not reported.

31. T.W. Meade, Sandra Dyer, Wendy Browne, Joy Townsend, and A.O. Frank, "Low Back Pain of Mechanical Origin: Randomised Comparison of Chiropractic and Hospital Outpatient Treatment," *British Medical Journal* (June 2, 1990): 1431–37; reprint in *Journal of Chiropractic* 27 (August 1990): 60–66, 68–69. Meade et al. also noted the positive economic implications associated with chiropractic care (vis-à-vis traditional hospital treatment) for low-back pain. See also "Low Back Pain: The Scorecard," *Harvard Medical School Health Letter* (September 1990): 1–2.

32. Rolland A. Martin, "A Study of Time Loss Back Claims," Workmen's Compensation Board, State of Oregon, March 1971, pp. 1, 3 (typescript).

33. C. Richard Wolf, "Industrial Back Injury," December 1972, Plaintiff's Exhibit No. 194, February 14, 1978, Wilk et al.: Complaint #76C3777. In addition, workmen's compensation studies in Florida (1961), Kansas (1971), and Iowa (for 1966 and 1969) show substantially less cost associated with chiropractic versus medical care of back injury. See R.C. Schafer, ed., *Chiropractic Health Care: A Conservative Approach to Health Restoration, Maintenance, and Disease Resistance,* 2d ed. (Des Moines, Iowa: Foundation for Chiropractic Education & Research, 1977), 86.

34. Robert L. Kane, Craig Leymaster, Donna Olsen, F. Ross Woolley, and F. David Fisher, "Manipulating the Patient: A Comparison of the Effectiveness of Physician and Chiropractic Care," *Lancet* (June 29, 1974): 1333–36. This study casts doubt on the often-expressed notion that chiropractors thrive by treating patients of low social and economic status, since the Utah State Insurance Fund (Workmen's Compensation) allows injured workers to choose their own practitioners. It also provides an example of direct competition between physicians and chiropractors.

35. Herbert H. Davis to [Silverman Chiropractic Center], March 9, 1983, Files, Law Offices of Allegretti, Newitt, Witcoff & McAndrews, Ltd., 125 South Wacker Drive, Chicago, Illinois. AV-MED headquarters are in Miami, Florida.

36. "Study of the First 100 Patients Referred to the Silverman Chiropractic Center by AV-MED," AV-MED Health Plan, Miami, Fla., n.d., c. 1984 (typescript). AV-MED polled these patients by telephone (reaching ninety-seven) about the results of their treatment. For each patient, the report gives the age, total cost, total number of chiropractic visits, number of physicians seen before and after chiropractic care, and comments on condition before and after treatment. According to "Chiropractic: State of the Art" (p. 3), seventy-five health plans included chiropractic manpower by the mid-1980s.

37. "What You Should Know about Chiropractic" (American Chiropractic Association, n.d., c. 1982), 3, 14–15; "Chiropractic: State of the Art," 1–3.

38. The two pieces in *Consumer's Report* became embroiled in the Wilk case controversy (see next section) when the plaintiffs charged that writer Joseph Botta had been duped by hostile propaganda and misinformation fed to him by the defendant AMA. Both plaintiffs and defendants sought discovery of Botta's sources while the Consumers Union (publishers of *Consumer's Report*) sought to quash subpoenas that would force them to divulge their sources and evaluation procedures. For the involved decision that partly granted and partly denied the motion to quash, see Consumers Union of United States, Inc., 495 F. Supp. 582 (1980).

The March 1981 *FDA Consumer* also carried a negative article ("Public Disservice Announcement," p. 32), but its wrath was directed not at chiropractic as a healing art, but at the Taylor Chiropractic Center for placing in a metropolitan Detroit newspaper an ad that had blasted the concept of immunization.

39. The other plaintiffs were James W. Bryden, Patricia A. Arthur, Steven G. Lumsden, and Michael D. Pedigo. Additional defendants were the American College of Surgeons, the American College of Physicians, the Joint Commission on Accreditation of Hospitals, the American College of Radiology, the Illinois State Medical Society, H. Doyl Taylor, Joseph A. Sabatier, M.D., H. Thomas Ballantine, M.D., and James H. Sammons, M.D. See Wilk v. American Medical Association, 719 F.2d 207 (7th Cir. 1983).

This was not the first time the AMA had been charged with violations of the Sherman Act. In American Medical Association v. United States, 317 U.S. 519 (1943), the Supreme Court upheld the ruling of the Court of Appeals, which had rejected the AMA's argument that antitrust laws do not apply to medicine because it is a profession rather than a trade. For discussion of the case, see Starr, *Social Transformation of American Medicine*, 305.

40. Sharon A. Christie, "Denial of Hospital Admitting Privileges for Non-Physician Providers—A Per Se Antitrust Violation?" *Notre Dame Law Review* 60 (Summer 1985): 725–26.

41. Wilk v. AMA, 719 F.2d at 208–9, 220–21. The Court of Appeals explained (p. 209) that section 1 of the Sherman Act, 15 U.S.C.A., section 1, allows the rule of reason test (under which the single standard is whether or not a challenged agreement promotes or suppresses competition) to be modified in antitrust cases involving the ethics of the medical profession. For a concise, legal discussion of this aspect of the case, see Christie, "Denial of Hospital Admitting Privileges," 741–42 n. 100. Christie argued (p. 737) that the patient care justification is "inappropriate in the context of blanket denial of [hospital] admitting privileges to non-physicians" and that (p. 738) "blanket denials of admitting privileges to non-physicians do not have a pro-competitive purpose."

Timothy Stoltzfus Jost, "The Joint Commission on Accreditation of Hospitals: Private Regulation of Health Care and the Public Interest," *Boston College Law Review* 24 (July 1983), argued (p. 873) that "many of these [non-M.D.] practitioners may need access to hospitals for certain aspects of their practice if they are to compete with physicians" and that (p. 908) "per se analysis might be appropriate both for analyzing the effects of JCAH on the competitors of its physician constituency and the competitors of its hospital constituency."

George P. McAndrews, "Non-Medical Physician Access: The Use of Anti-trust Concepts to Overcome Anti-Competitive Barriers," paper presented before the National Health Lawyers Association, Washington, D.C., January 23–25, 1985, provided an important overview of the subject.

By mid-1985, some chiropractic groups had begun a concerted effort to gain hospital admitting privileges. See California Chiropractic Association, "Hospital Privileges Kit," June 1985 (typescript).

42. Brief for Plaintiffs-Appellants at 11 and 12, Wilk v. AMA, 719 F.2d 207 (7th Cir. 1983) (No. 81-1331), cert. denied, 104 S.Ct. 2398 (1984).

43. Confidential memorandum from the Committee on Quackery to the AMA Board of Trustees, January 4, 1971, quoted in Wilk v. AMA 719 F.2d at 213. The memorandum also noted: "Your Committee believes it is well along with its first mission and is, at the same time, moving toward the ultimate goal. This, then might be considered a progress report on developments in the past seven years. The Committee has not previously submitted such a report because it believes that to make public some of its activities would have been and continues to be unwise. Thus, this report is intended only for the information of the Board of Trustees." Defendants Drs. Ballantine and Sabatier were chairmen of the committee and defendant Doyl Taylor, formerly a sports editor of the *Des Moines Register* whose brother was the executive director of the Iowa Medical Society, was secretary. Throckmorton had brought Taylor to the AMA in Chicago to work on the plan. The other individual defendant, Dr. Sammons, was executive vice-president of the AMA and as a member of the AMA Board of Trustees approved the goals, operations, and funding of the Committee on Quackery.

44. Brief for Plaintiffs-Appellants at 16–18; Wilk v. AMA, 719 F.2d at 213. Principle 4 of the code states: "Physicians . . . should expose, without hesitation, . . . unethical conduct of fellow members of the profession." Any association with chiropractors was now, by definition, unethical.

45. Brief for Plaintiffs-Appellants at 18; Wilk v. AMA, 719 F.2d at 213, 214; "Finally . . . Guilty!!!" (Huntington Beach, Calif.: Motion Palpation Institute, 1987), 6.

46. Otto Arndal, Director, Hospital Accreditation Program to Norman H. Meyer, Administrator, Hillcrest General Hospital [Silver City, New Mexico], January 9, 1973, Plaintiffs' Exhibit 10A, transcribed in Brief for Plaintiffs-Appellants at 19. See also Henry K. Speed, Jr., Associate Director [JCAH] to Sister Daniel Marie, Administrator, St. Joseph Hospital [Stanford, Conn.], April 5, 1974, Plaintiffs' Exhibit 11A, and Speed to Hans A. Dahl, Administrator, Rice Memorial Hospital [Willmar, Minn.], August 13, 1974. Plaintiffs' Exhibit 14A, transcribed in Brief at 20.

47. Plaintiffs' Exhibits 1354, 353, 72, cited in Brief at 18, 22. See also "Victory!" *Dynamic Chiropractic* 5 (September 15, 1987): 3.

48. Wilk v. AMA, 671 F. Supp. at 1465, 1477–78, 1506 (N.D. Ill. 1987). See also, "Wilk Wins: AMA Found Guilty in Eleven-Year Old Anti-Trust Suit," *The Chiropractic Journal* 2 (October 1987): 1, 9, and "Victory!" 3, 38–39.

49. Wilk v. AMA, 671 F. Supp. at 1488. The article mentioned by Getzendanner appeared in *JAMA* 226 (November 12, 1973): 829–30.

50. Wilk v. AMA, 671 F. Supp. at 1507–8; "Finally . . . Guilty!!!" 18–19; *Roanoke Times & World News,* April 22, 1990.

51. "Wilk Wins," 9.

52. Leigh Page, "*Wilk* Ruling Could Ease Restrictions on Chiropractic," *American Medical News* (December 11, 1987): 3.

53. "Statement on Interprofessional Relations with Doctors of Chiropractic," *Illinois Medical Journal* 167 (April 1985): 273. See also Howard Wolinsky, "Ruling Allows Chiropractors to Practice with Physicians," *Chicago Sun-Times,* March 5, 1985, and Ronald Koltulak, "Chiropractors, Doctors at Peace: They'll Work Together," *Chicago Tribune,* March 5, 1985.

54. The Detroit ad and Gray are quoted in Mark Holoweiko, "The New Health-Care Partnership: M.D.'s and D.C.'s" *Medical Economics* (May 27, 1985): 81, 82. See also Eileen Keerdoja et al., "A New Medical Marriage," *Newsweek* (August 12, 1985): 69, 71.

CHAPTER SEVEN. POETRY WITH SCIENCE: THE FLOURISHING OF CHIROPRACTIC

1. For example, Arthur Wrobel, ed., *Pseudo-Science and Society in Nineteenth-Century America* (Lexington, Ky.: University Press of Kentucky, 1987), and Meredith B. McGuire, "The New Spirituality: Healing Rituals Hit the Suburbs," *Psychology Today* (January–February 1989): 57–64, do not include chiropractic. Reporting on a survey published initially in the May 1989 *American Journal of Public Health,* the July 1989 *Medical Abstracts Newsletter* (p. 2) noted that only 3 percent of 489 family physicians surveyed in the state of Washington "dismissed chiropractors as quacks that patients should avoid."

2. Quoted in Perry Miller, *Jonathan Edwards* (New York: William Sloane Associates, 1949), 234.

3. Paul C. Reisser, Teri K. Reisser, and John Weldon, *New Age Medicine* (Downers Grove, Ill.: InterVarsity Press, 1987), 87–89.

4. Patrick Cooke, "The Crescent City Cure," *Hippocrates* (November–December 1988): 60–70.

5. Reisser, Reisser, and Weldon, *New Age Medicine,* 142–46, 19–20, 80–87. Evangelical Christians have raised the concern that chiropractic harbors dangers through association with New Age medical practices that have metaphysical underpinnings derived from Eastern mysticism (see ibid., also pp. 176–77 n.1). Most current chiropractors, however, seem to downplay if not shun the metaphysical roots of the discipline. Evangelicals seem to be unaware that, even though the Palmer ideology has certain affinities to Eastern mysticism with its direction of unseen life forces and energies, it is more clearly a popular manifestation of the Western harmonial tradition.

6. John Naisbitt, *Megatrends: Ten New Directions Transforming Our Lives* (New York: Warner Books, 1982), 48, 39.

7. "Round Table: Survival Tactics for the Jungle Out There," *Medical Economics* (May 30, 1983): 72.

8. Medical doctors are becoming increasingly aware of their deficiencies in these areas. See H.G. Whittington, "We Can Learn from Non-M.D. Healers—and We'd Better," *Medical Economics* (October 17, 1983): 84, 87. Merrijoy Kelner, Oswald Hall, and Ian Coulter, in *Chiropractors: Do They Help?* (Toronto: Fitzhenry & Whiteside, 1980), 82–83, pointed out that chiropractic education is directed

toward a general, solo practice, encouraging "the development of a personal style of interaction between future practitioners and the patients with whom they come in contact," permitting "students to take a positive, holistic attitude toward the health problems they encounter." In sharp contrast, "the current medical approach to selecting recruits seems to favor the selection of highly competitive, academically skillful, science-oriented persons for what is essentially a people-oriented profession."

Some mainstream medical people are now touting a technique known as "therapeutic touch"—a concept that sounds remarkably akin to D.D. Palmer's magnetic healing and early chiropractic ideology. It is defined as "a method of facilitating healing in which a universal life energy is channelled through one individual to another. It is based on the belief that a human being is a complex energy pattern and that disease represents congestion and imbalance in this pattern." From the brochure advertising the "Holistic Nursing Workshop: Therapeutic Touch," April 29, 1989, Continuing Education, College of Nursing, Clemson University, convening to aid nurses, physicians, therapists, counselors, and other allied health professionals. Topics on the agenda included meditation, guided imagery, guided fantasy, Kirlian photography, personal space, energy fields, unruffling the field, and knowing when to stop. See also Lynn Agoglia Miller, "An Explanation of Therapeutic Touch: Using the Science of Unitary Man," *Nursing Forum* 18 (1979): 278–87.

9. It is a common notion that success achieved by any alternative therapy can be explained by the placebo effect. This idea falls especially short when applied to chiropractic because a large percentage of patients through the years have gone for adjustments as a last resort armed with great skepticism. The placebo effect operates on the premise that the patient believes that the treatment will be effective; skepticism sqelches success. Therapeutic success under such conditions cannot be ascribed to the placebo. Once a patient becomes convinced of the value of chiropractic, a placebo effect could perhaps begin to operate. For a typical statement that chiropractic works because of the placebo effect, see a report cited in Marshall W. Raffel, *The U.S. Health System: Origins and Functions*, 2d ed. (New York: John Wiley & Sons, 1980), 150.

10. Palmer quoted in Gielow, *Old Dad Chiro*, 109–10. In "Homeopathic Chic," Mary Carpenter (*Health*, March 1989, p. 93) discussed the *esprit frondeur* as a reason for the recent revival of homeopathy in France. The phrase comes from the *Fronde*, a French political party organized during the seventeenth century to oppose the court and Cardinal Jules Mazarin.

Particular articles in the press also galvanized chiropractors. Martha Metz (*Fifty Years of Chiropractic*, 88–89) noted a hostile piece in *Reader's Digest* that "served to unite [chiropractic] factions in the common cause of resisting the enemy."

11. Whorton, *Crusaders for Fitness*, 167.

12. Whorton himself made no connection between chiropractic and these particular ideas. Samuel Hopkins Adams's *The Clarion* (Boston: Houghton Mifflin Co., 1914) is an interesting fictional treatment of the downfall of Dr. L. Andre Surtaine, vendor of the nostrum Certina, which clearly illustrates the Progressive suspicion of drugs.

13. In 1985, the Bureau of Labor Statistics noted that the number of

chiropractors could double by 1995, raising the total to some sixty thousand. See Carol Kleiman, "Chiro Ranks to Double by 1995," *Moline Dispatch,* June 17, 1985.

14. Quoted in Fishbein, *Fads and Quackery in Healing,* 242.

POSTSCRIPT: PROSPECTS FOR THE FUTURE OF CHIROPRACTIC

1. For example, a recent article in the *Roanoke [Va.] Times & World News* ("Back in Shape," May 16, 1991) discussed the various types of specialists who treat back pain and noted that "perhaps the most controversial specialist is the chiropractor. While many people swear by them, surgeons and physicians have long been skeptical about the efficacy and even the safety of spinal manipulation."

2. Martin S. Pernick, *A Calculus of Suffering: Pain, Professionalism, and Anesthesia in Nineteenth-Century America* (New York: Columbia University Press, 1985), 242. Pernick brought a refreshing and much-needed clarity to the sometimes bewildering array of material on professionalism. See esp. pp. 214–48.

3. Walter I. Wardwell, "The Present and Future Role of the Chiropractor," in *Modern Developments in the Principles and Practices of Chiropractic,* ed. Scott Haldeman (New York: Appleton-Century-Crofts, 1980), 40–41. Wardwell has a new book out entitled *Chiropractic: History and Evolution of a New Profession* (St. Louis: Mosby-Year Book, 1992), which appeared while this book was in press.

4. *The Chiropractic Journal* 2 (October 1987): 7.

5. "Attorney George P. McAndrews Responds to Drs. Jarvis and Barrett," *Journal of Chiropractic* 27 (August 1990): 48.

6. Richard H. Tyler, "Hospitals and the Real Protocol for Chiropractors," *Dynamic Chiropractic* 5 (September 15, 1987): 41.

7. In "The Need for Chiropractic Research," *Today's Chiropractic* 19 (July–August 1990): 89, Randy Southerland noted that "increased scientific respectability has meant greater acceptance in the medical marketplace. Chiropractors are beginning to take their places as directors of chiropractic departments in hospitals, for example. Observers agree that this trend is likely to continue, as research makes it increasingly difficult to attach the 'quack' label to practitioners."

Bibliographical Essay

Perspectives on Healing, Orthodoxy, and Chiropractic

Of all the nations of the world, the United States is most afflicted by its healers. Besides those holding the degree M.D., signifying doctor of medicine and, nowadays, some seven years of study following high school graduation, a host of queer practitioners pervade the medical field. They have conferred on themselves strange combinations of letters, indicating the peculiar systems of healing which a somewhat lax system of legislation and law enforcement permits them to practice on an unwary public.

Morris Fishbein, *Fads and Quackery in Healing*

Doctors are whippersnappers in ironed white coats
Who spy up your rectums and look down your throats
And press you and poke you with sterilized tools
And stab at solutions that pacify fools.
I used to revere them and do what they said
Till I learned what they learned on was already dead.

Gilda Radner, "Doctors Are Whippersnappers,"
The New England Journal of Medicine

"Queer practitioners" are queer only because they advocate principles and procedures distinctly different from the dominant medical group who determine, at any given time, the boundaries of orthodox or "regular" medicine. Regular doctors themselves have suffered a checkered reputation throughout American history, which has given rise to a succession of irregular practitioners and apostles of self-help. But not all of those who have counseled against medical care for illness have done so primarily because they hold the medical profession in low esteem. For example, Ronald L. Numbers pointed out in *Prophetess of Health* (New York: Harper & Row, 1976) that Ellen G. White, noted Adventist prophetess of the nineteenth century, believed that consulting physicians constituted a denial of faith and charged her flock to seek the healing power of God by laying hold of the promises of James 5:14–15 and avoid "applying to earthly physicians."

Even in a late twentieth-century America booming with CT scanners and chemotherapeutic "magic bullets" that exude an aura of scientific mastery, unorthodox healers and techniques still thrive as ever-present testimony to the limits of modern medicine. A stroll through any commercial bookstore reveals shelves bulging with "New Age" health titles such as *Crystal Clear: How to Use the Earth's Magic Energy to Vitalize Your Body, Mind, and Spirit* (complete with plastic casing holding a quartz crystal designed as an aid to "Harmonize, Vitalize, Realize Your Mind, Body, Spirit"); *The Women's Book of Healing: Auras & Laying on of Hands, Crystals & Gemstones, Chakras & Colors; The New Holistic Health Handbook: Living Well in a New Age; The New Astrology; The New Book of Runes; Selective Awareness: Discover Your Infinite Potential for Self-Healing and Growth; The Creative Visualization Workbook;* and *The Heart of Zen Cuisine.* Mainstream publications as diverse as *Time* magazine ("New Age Harmonies," a cover story on December 7, 1987), *Psychology Today* ("The New Spirituality: Healing Rituals Hit the Suburbs," January–February 1989), and *Women's World* ("Nature's Clinic: Can Crystals Really Heal?" May 31, 1988) have all chronicled a burgeoning interest in alternative therapies that tap into the spirit of the ancient hermetic tradition and the more recent harmonial tradition. On hermeticism, see A.-J. Festugiere, *La revelation d'Hermes Trismegiste,* 4 vols. (Paris, Librairie Lecoffre, 1949–54); Frances A. Yates, *Giordano Bruno and the Hermetic Tradition* (Chicago: University of Chicago Press, 1964); D.P. Walker, *The Ancient Theology: Studies in Christian Platonism from the Fifteenth Century to the Eighteenth Century* (Ithaca, N.Y.: Cornell University Press, 1972); Wayne Shumaker, *The Occult Sciences in the Renaissance: A Study in Intellectual Patterns* (Berkeley and Los Angeles: University of California Press, 1972); Garth Fowden, *The Egyptian Hermes: A Historical Approach to the Late Pagan Mind* (Cambridge: Cambridge University Press, 1986); Ingrid Merkel and Allen G. Debus, eds., *Hermeticism and the Renaissance: Intellectual History and the Occult in Early Modern Europe* (Washington: Folger Shakespeare Library, 1988).

On the American harmonial tradition see Robert C. Fuller, *Alternative Medicine and American Religious Life* (New York: Oxford University Press, 1989); Donald Meyer, *The Positive Thinkers: Religion as Pop Psychology from Mary Baker Eddy to Oral Roberts,* 2d ed. (New York: Pantheon, 1980); Sydney E. Ahlstrom, *A Religious History of the American People* (New Haven:

Yale University Press, 1972), esp. 1019–36. Ahlstrom noted (p. 1038) that hermeticism is closely akin to American developments (such as Theosophy) that lie outside the Judeo-Christian tradition.

The historical persistence of nonorthodox "-pathies" and "-ologies" suggests an important social and intellectual as well as medical phenomenon of more than antiquarian or pedantic interest. Orthodoxy is ever-shifting, sometimes crawling in small, barely noticeable increments, sometimes in easily discernible leaps. Heterodox movements help determine the directions of orthodoxy, as well as the reverse.

Traditionally, those who have written about heterodox healing movements have either taken the perspective of medical orthodoxy, producing tirades against the movements, or upheld alternative therapies, penning polemics accusing detractors of shortsightedness and self-interest. Typically, medical doctors have taken the perspective of orthodoxy, embracing a Whig interpretation of medical progress that views the heterodox healer as a temporary, pseudoscientific nuisance to be hustled from the path of a forward-marching, genuinely scientific medicine. Morris Fishbein's work denouncing medical fads of the 1920s and 1930s well illustrates the perspective. "After all," he explained in *Fads and Quackery in Healing* (Chicago: n.p., 1932), "the progress of scientific medicine is a powerful movement sweeping on and on with ever increasing impetus. The 'fly on the chariot wheel' cannot halt it; but there is danger that the swarm of flies may impede its movement." This confident faith in the progress of medical orthodoxy was nothing new. Richard H. Shryock's essay on "Medical Sources and the Social Historian" in the *American Historical Review* of April 1936 noted that the first real attempt in medical historiography published in the United States (David Ramsey's *Review of the Improvements, Progress, and State of Medicine in the XVIIIth Century*, 1801) was typical of the era and that present readers might be surprised to learn that "eighteenth century writers were just as optimistic about 'the triumphs of modern medicine' as anyone is today." This Whig interpretation is still alive and well. Francis D. Moore, M.D., in a review of Sherwin Nuland's *Doctors: The Biography of Medicine* for *The New England Journal of Medicine* (November 17, 1988), took the opportunity to applaud Nuland for avoiding

> the preposterous errors of the socioeconomic and political theorists (e.g. Paul Starr in *The Social Transformation of American Medicine* . . .), who seem to believe that Western medicine won out over quacks and cults by political battling in some Chicago venue. It is perfectly clear that Western medicine, starting with the Renaissance, succeeded over cults and sorcery because it was based on scientific data and concepts that worked and were effective in sick people, and on the facts of biology as they were progressively uncovered. Diphtheria and tetanus antitoxins, clean surgery, and insulin were far more important than American Medical Association lawsuits.

On the other side, the advocacy perspective of the unorthodox has been argued most vigorously by the founders of the various systems and their zealous followers. They frequently charge the regulars themselves with quackery and charlatanry and promote their own therapies as much-needed reform, often undergirded with a new philosophical understanding. Samuel Thomson, originator of the popular botanic system in the early nineteenth century known as Thomsonianism, asked readers of his autobiography (quoted by Norman Gevitz, "Three Perspectives on Unorthodox Medicine," in *Other Healers: Unorthodox Medicine in America* [Baltimore: Johns Hopkins University Press, 1988], 17–18) to determine "which is the greatest quack, the one who relieves them from their sickness by the most simple and safe means, without any pretensions to infallibility or skill, more than what nature and experience has taught him; or the one who, instead of curing the disease, increases it by poisonous medicines which only tend to prolong the distress of the patient, till wither the strength of his natural constitution, or death relieves him." Twentieth-century advocates of alternative therapies such as Brian Inglis in *The Case for Unorthodox Medicine* (New York: Putnam, 1965) continue to echo Thomson, charging the medical establishment with responsibility for creating a drug-crazed society subject to chemically induced misery and death.

By the 1950s, another perspective was emerging, one that attempted to avoid the traditional saint-or-sinner polarity. Academically oriented researchers began employing a new scholarly perspective by using a wide array of sources, seeking to understand the phenomenon of unorthodox medicine in its social and cultural context and abandoning the intention of ferreting out falsehood and safeguarding truth that constrained prior studies. This independent perspective emphasized the ambiguities involved in determining healing effectiveness and helped free the study of unorthodox medicine from reliance on unexamined labels (such as quack, crank, and pseudoscientist) that frequently obscured rather than aided understanding.

Norman Gevitz's essay mentioned above ("Three Perspectives" in *Other Healers*) provides an excellent overview of the historiography of unorthodox medicine. For recent historiographical treatments of American medical history written from the scholarly perspective, see Ronald L. Numbers, "The History of American Medicine: A Field in Ferment," *Reviews in American History* 10 (December 1982): 245–63; Charles E. Rosenberg, "Bibliographical Note," in George Rosen, *The Structure of American Medical Practice, 1875–1941,* ed. Charles E. Rosenberg (Philadelphia, University of Pennsylvania Press, 1983), 141–46; and John Harley Warner, "Science in Medicine," *Osiris: A Research Journal Devoted to the History of Science and Its Cultural Influence,* 2d ser., 1 (1985): 37–58.

On the relationship among the Mind Cure, New Thought, and Christian Science movements see Donald Meyer, *The Positive Thinkers,* esp.

32–45, 73–93; John F. Teahan, "Warren Felt Evans and Mental Healing: Romantic Idealism and Practical Mysticism in Nineteenth-Century America," *Church History* 48 (March 1979): 63–80; Raymond J. Cunningham, "Christian Science and Mind Cure in America: A Review Article," *Journal of the History of the Behavioral Sciences* 11 (July 1975): 299–305.

Yet even scholarly treatments can too easily lapse into a smug, presentist use of labels. For example, articles in *Pseudo-Science and Society in Nineteenth-Century America,* ed. Arthur Wrobel (Lexington: University Press of Kentucky, 1987), sometimes assume a clear dichotomy between science and pseudoscience. All pseudoscience really means, as Henry Bauer has pointed out in *Beyond Velikovsky: The History of a Public Controversy* (Urbana: University of Illinois Press, 1984), is that something is outside the currently accepted bounds of science, not that the ideas involved are necessarily wrong. "In common usage nowadays," Bauer noted (p. 254), " 'scientific' is synonymous with 'true'; we habitually forget that science does not deal in absolute truth; we use semantic devices that obscure the distinction between science and truth; we talk as though they were one and the same thing."

William Rothstein, in his influential *American Physicians in the Nineteenth Century: From Sects to Science* (Baltimore: Johns Hopkins University Press, 1972), 23, defined a medical sect as consisting "of a number of physicians, together with their professional institutions, who utilize medically valid therapies when they exist, but otherwise utilize a distinctive set of medically invalid therapies rejected by other sects" and identified regulars in the nineteenth century as one among a number of competing sects. According to Rothstein, orthodox medicine emerged from the realms of sectarianism when it embraced "medically valid therapies" made available by modern science. This distinction, however, between "valid" and "invalid" therapies is much too positivistic and assumes that a clear distinction is easily made.

Scholars took up study of the nonorthodox from the independent perspective and soon demonstrated the value of understanding "deviant" theories and therapies from outside the movements. In *The Positive Thinkers,* Donald Meyer traced the various strains of the mind-cure movements from Mary Baker Eddy to the health-and-wealth therapists of our own day. Ronald Numbers in *Prophetess of Health* (mentioned above) examined the healing messages of Adventist prophetess Ellen G. White and the spiritual meaning of healing, while Steven Nissenbaum explored the environment of health reform in the nineteenth century by focusing on Sylvester Graham in *Sex, Diet, and Debility in Jacksonian America* (Westport, Conn.: Greenwood Press, 1980). Sarah Stage studied the patent medicine business of Lydia Pinkham in *Female Complaints* (New York: W.W. Norton, 1979) as a pathway to understanding women's health at the turn of the century, and

James Whorton sought to balance the comic stature of nineteenth-century health fanatics by understanding the serious aspects of their reforms and the spiritual context of their crusades in *Crusaders for Fitness: The History of American Health Reformers* (Princeton: Princeton University Press, 1982). Most recently, Robert Fuller in *Alternative Medicine and American Religious Life* (cited above) has clarified how religious impulses informed and directed alternative medical movements in America.

James Harvey Young made scholarly attempts to investigate individual "quacks" without *intentional* malice toward the individuals or the particular groups they represent in *The Toadstool Millionaires: A Social History of Patent Medicines in America before Federal Regulation* (Princeton: Princeton University Press, 1961) and *The Medical Messiahs: A Social History of Health Quackery in Twentieth-Century America* (Princeton, 1967). Gerald Carson provided a colorful account of John Harvey Kellogg and the burgeoning health food business in *Cornflake Crusade* (New York: Rinehart & Co., 1957). On domestic medicine, see Guenter B. Risse, Ronald L. Numbers, and Judith Walzer Leavitt, eds., *Medicine without Doctors: Home Health Care in American History* (New York: Science History Publications, 1977), and Anita Clair Fellman and Michael Fellman, *Making Sense of Self: Medical Advice Literature in Late Nineteenth-Century America* (Philadelphia: University of Pennsylvania Press, 1981).

Other scholars began to reevaluate the major alternative groups in book-length treatments. Martin Kaufman provided a comprehensive and balanced view of homeopathy as a "medical heresy" in *Homeopathy in America* (Baltimore: Johns Hopkins University Press, 1971), and Norman Gevitz in *The D.O.'s* (Baltimore: Johns Hopkins University Press, 1982) offered a scholarly portrait of osteopathy. Both Jane Donegan (*Hydropathic Highway to Health: Women and Water-Cure in Antebellum America* [Westport, Conn.: Greenwood Press, 1986]) and Susan Cayleff (*"Wash and Be Healed": The Water-Cure Movement and Women's Health* [Philadelpha: Temple University Press, 1987]) have accounted for the rise of the water cure (hydropathy) in mid-nineteenth century America, adding to the earlier work of Harry Weiss and Howard Kemble in *The Great American Water-Cure Craze: A History of Hydropathy in the United States* (Trenton, N.J.: Past Times Press, 1967). Curiously, the largest of all the alternative American movements—chiropractic—has received only the most cursory treatment from medical historians. In 1932, Morris Fishbein wrote in *Fads and Quackery in Healing* that "just what the ultimate outcome of the chiropractic cult will be no one knows." Now we have a much clearer picture. Unlike the other nonorthodox medical movements of the nineteenth century, chiropractic has not only survived intact, but also flourished. Chiropractic is now the second largest healing group in America (after medical doctors) and the most widespread drugless therapy in the world. Chiropractic occupies a unique place among alternative healers. Growing out of the late nineteenth century, it followed a path typical of medical sectarianism—charismatic leaders with self-proclaimed divine inspiration, miraculous and immediate cures of apparently hopeless conditions, zealous true believers as followers, irreconcilable schisms, intense and repeated persecutions, battles with the law—all except the inevitable oblivion or absorption suffered by other movements. It could perhaps be argued that Christian Science has also flourished; between 1900 and 1915, however, as Rennie B. Schoepflin noted ("Christian Science Healing in America," in *Other Healers*, 207), "the changing attitude of the courts toward the control and regulation of medical practice drove Scientists from the school of medicine to the sanctuary of religion, and [Mary Baker] Eddy's own experience hastened the Journey." Other "generic" Christian Scientists, holdovers from the New Thought movement such as Unity, Religious Science, and Divine Science, are also primarily religious rather than medical movements. By 1985, there were 2,884 Christian Science practitioners in the United States (Schoepflin, p. 212). By the mid-1980s, there were some thirty-five thousand chiropractors, and the numbers have continued to grow.

Because chiropractic sprang from sources common to cultism and yet avoided the common fate, the flourishing of chiropractic represents an important social and medical phenomenon. "Whatever its merits, or even whether it has any or not," Samuel Grafton recognized in "The Case for Chiropractic," (*McCall's*, October 1959), chiropractic "is, because of its persistence and growth, probably deserving of more serious social study, if only as a phenomenon, than it has received. But most of the literature on the subject is either outright praise or outright abuse."

Thirty years later, the situation is little changed. Just as medical doctors traditionally wrote medical history from the orthodox perspective, chiropractors have written chiropractic history from the vantage of the nonorthodox, countered periodically by establishment writers who indignantly demanded excision of the "malignant tumor" of chiropractic (Morris Fishbein's diagnosis in *Fads and Quackery*, p. 86) from the body of scientific medicine. Another but somewhat less vociferous example of this viewpoint is Louis Reed's in *The Healing Cults: A Study of Sectarian Medical Practice* (Chicago: University of Chicago Press, 1932). Ralph Lee Smith's polemic *At Your Own Risk: The Case against Chiropractic* (New York: Trident Press, 1969) is a particularly vicious assault that argues for repeal of chiropractic licensure laws.

Consigned to an aberrant role by the orthodox, chiropractors developed a ghetto mentality that has pushed them, in defense, to produce more hagiology than history. Typical of this effort is A. Augustus Dye's assessment of D.D. Palmer, the originator of chiropractic, in *The Evolution of Chiropractic* (Philadelphia: by the author, 1939): "For D.D. was not a man to swerve from his path, once he had started a journey, convinced he was going the right way. His desire was to see chiropractic reach its ultimate destiny unmixed with elements and practices purloined from other healing systems" (p. 15). More recently, Joseph E. Maynard, D.C., echoed this perspective in *Healing Hands: The Story of the Palmer Family, Discoverers of Chiropractic* (Mobile, Ala.: Jonorm Publishers, 1959, rev. ed., 1977).

> Without Daniel David Palmer, the discoverer, this scientific method of correcting the cause of dis-ease by hand may never have been developed to save the lives of so many sick, medically-disappointed, people.
>
> It took an uninhibited individualist, an intellect whose mind could accept a radical, "new" idea; it took a strong, determined man who could not be defeated by the scorn of his fellows, by the clogged, rusty-thinking of so-called "scientists." It took a pioneer. . . .
>
> And it took D.D. Palmer's son, Bartlett Joshua Palmer, the apostle of this new science, to take up where his father left off and fight those who sought to stop Man from benefiting from Chiropractic.
>
> He fought and he won.

Other treatments from the chiropractic perspective include D.D. Palmer's own *Text-Book of the Science, Art and Philosophy of Chiropractic, for Students and Practitioners* (Portland, Oreg.: Portland Printing House, 1910); the so-called Palmer "Green Books," a series of some thirty-nine erratically numbered volumes (most with dark green binding) printed by the Palmer School, many penned by B.J. Palmer in a stream-of-consciousness style (see Glenda C. Wiese and Michelle R. Lykins, "The Palmer Green Books, Volume 1, 1906–Volume 39, 1966: An Annotated Bibliography," May 1986, typescript, Palmer College of Chiropractic Archives, Davenport, Iowa, and Wiese and Lykins, "A Bibliography of the Palmer Green Books in Print, 1906–1985," *Chiropractic History: The Archives and Journal of the Association for the History of Chiropractic* 6 [1986]: 65–74); Harry Gallaher, D.C., *History of Chiropractic: A History of the Philosophy, Art and Science of Chiropractic and Chiropractors in Oklahoma Together with a Biographical History of the Prominent Exponents of the Science in Oklahoma* (Guthrie, Okla.: William E. Welch & William H. Pattie, 1930); Chittenden Turner, *The Rise of Chiropractic* (Los Angeles: Powell Publishing Co., 1931); Martha M. Metz, D.C., *Fifth Years of Chiropractic Recognized in Kansas* (Abilene, Kans.: Shadinger-Wilson, 1965); Sol Goldschmidt, D.C., "A Brief History of Chiropractic in New York State, 1902–1963," (n.p.: New York State Chiropractic Association, [1965]); Marcus Bach, *The Chiropractic Story* (Austell, Ga.: Si-Nel Publishing & Sales Co., 1968); Chester A. Wilk, D.C., *Chiropractic Speaks Out: A Reply to Medical Propaganda, Bigotry and Ignorance* (Park Ridge, Ill.: Wilk Publishing Co., 1973); Walter R. Rhodes, *The Official History of Chiropractic in Texas* (Austin: Texas Chiropractic Association, 1978); Vern Gielow, *Old Dad Chiro: A*

Biography of D.D. Palmer, Founder of Chiropractic (Davenport, Iowa: Bawden Bros., 1981); and R.B. Mawhiney, D.C., *Chiropractic in Wisconsin, 1900–1950* (n.p.: Wisconsin Chiropractic Association, 1984).

One enigmatic unpublished source, the so-called Lerner Report, merits special mention. In 1952, a New York lawyer named Cyrus Lerner was commissioned by the Foundation for Health Research, a chiropractic organization dominated by pro-B.J. members, to record the early history of the profession by interviewing B.J. and his associates. Apparently, the Palmers were distraught by a number of Lerner's interpretations, especially one that described B.J. as a "multiple personality." According to the archivist of Palmer College (in our conversation on August 1, 1986), B.J.'s son Dave suppressed the Lerner Report and ordered copies burned. She told me that the archives had no copy. However, several writers in *Chiropractic History* have cited the Lerner Report in their articles, noting the Palmer College Archives as their source. One writer (in an article published in 1981) cited the Lyndon E. Lee Papers in the Palmer Archives as the specific source. Lee was a member of the Foundation for Health Research and his papers contain a letter from B.J. (June 21, 1952) giving his approval for the project and a letter from Dave Palmer (June 30, 1969) indicating Palmer's attempt to acquire the Lerner material. A June 23, 1972, letter from Dave Palmer to Lee makes it clear that the material had indeed arrived in Davenport, "stored in my vault so that they're absolutely safe from fire, vandalism, theft, etc., to be perpetuated for someone who someday, sometime, will have the time to put together a fascinating history of the early struggles and trials of the profession." The Lerner Report seems to have led an underground existence, available only to the chiropractic fraternity until very recently. In response to my further inquiry, the Palmer archivist wrote (in a letter dated June 30, 1988) that the Lerner Report "was sent to us as part of the Lyndon Lee papers" after my research trip (in the summer of 1986). When I was in Davenport during that summer, I did find in the Lee Papers the intriguing, annotated "Topical Index" to the report, which contains a number of valuable insights.

In *The True Believer: Thoughts on the Nature of Mass Movements* (New York: Harper & Row, 1951), sociologist Eric Hoffer argued that the "true believer," whether writer, artist, or scientist, does not create to discover "the true and the beautiful" but rather "to warn, to advise, to urge, to glorify and to denounce" (p. 140). Even though true believers have written most chiropractic history, the value of the information presented and the insight provided into the character of a heterodox medical movement should not be dismissed or trivialized. But the perspective and intention of these writers should be clearly understood, as should the intention of those who attempt to deflate chiropractic from the Olympian perspective of "medical science," an outlook that can also easily assume the viewpoint of a true believer. Bernie Siegel suggested in *Love, Medicine & Miracles* (New York: Harper & Row, 1986) that "all healing is scientific" (p. 129) and "that one generation's miracle may be another's scientific fact" (p. 6).

Only recently have glimmers of a scholarly perspective on chiropractic history begun to emerge. Both Russell Gibbons and sociologist Walter Wardwell treated various aspects of chiropractic from an independent standpoint, but Gibbons himself recently lamented the absence of any "real history" of chiropractic survival ("The Evolution of Chiropractic: Medical and Social Protest in America, Notes on the Survival Years and After," in *Modern Developments in the Principles and Practice of Chiropractic,* ed. Scott Haldeman [New York: Appleton-Century-Crofts, 1980], 5). Gibbons's other articles include "Physician-Chiropractors: Medical Presence in the Evolution of Chiropractic," *Bulletin of the History of Medicine* 55 (Summer 1981): 233–45; "Chiropractic: Conflicts in Cultism and Science," paper presented at the 1977 annual meeting of the Popular Culture Association, Baltimore, Maryland, April 29, 1977 (typescript); "Chiropractic in America: The Historical Conflicts of Cultism and Science," *The Journal of Popular Culture* 10 (1977): 720–31; "Solon Massey Langworthy: Keeper of the Flame during the 'Lost Years' of Chiropractic," *Chiropractic History* 1 (1981): 15–21; "Forgotten Perameters [*sic*] of General Practice: The Chiropractic Obstetrician," *Chiropractic History* 2 (1982): 27–33; "Chiropractors as Interns, Residents and Staff: The Hospital Experience, 1910–1960," *Chiropractic History* 3 (1983): 51–57; "Chiropractic's Abraham Flexner: The Lonely Journey of John J. Nugent, 1935–1963," *Chiropractic History* 5 (1985): 44–51; "Assessing the Oracle at the Fountainhead: B.J. Palmer and His Times, 1902–1961," *Chiropractic History* 7 (July 1987): 8–14; "The Rise of the Chiropractic Educational Establishment, 1897–1980," in *Who's Who in Chiropractic International,* 2d ed., ed. Fern Lints-Dzaman (Littleton, Colo.: Who's Who in Chiropractic International Publishing Co., 1980), 339–52. Gibbons's efforts are highly competent but occasionally fall into what I would call the in-house, scholarly perspective—a vantage point that remains independent but sometimes loses sight of the larger context by revolving around the interior workings of the subject to such an extent that it can take on an antiquarian hue.

Wardwell's significant contribution to the field includes "Social Strain and Social Adjustment in the Marginal Role of the Chiropractor" (Ph.D. diss., Harvard University, 1951); "A Marginal Professional Role: The Chiropractor," *Social Forces* 30 (1952): 339–48; "The Reduction of Strain in a Marginal Role," *American Journal of Sociology* 61 (1955): 16–26; "Limited, Marginal and Quasi-Practitioners," in *Handbook of Medical Sociology,* eds. Howard Freeman, Sol Levine, and Leo Reeder (Englewood Cliffs, N.J.: Prentice Hall Press, 1963), 213–39, 2d ed., 1972, pp. 250–73; "Discussion: The Impact of Spinal Manipulative Therapy on the Health

Care System," in U.S. Department of Health, Education, and Welfare, Public Health Service, National Institutes of Health, and the National Institute of Neurological and Communicative Disorders and Stroke Cooperating, *The Research Status of Spinal Manipulative Therapy: A Workshop Held at the National Institutes of Health, February 2–4, 1975*, ed. Murray Goldstein, DHEW publication no. (NIH) 76-998, pp. 53–58; "Social Factors in the Survival of Chiropractic: A Comparative View," *Sociological Symposium* (Spring 1978): 6–17; "The Present and Future Role of the Chiropractor," in *Modern Developments in the Principles and Practices of Chiropractic*, 25–41; "The Cutting Edge of Chiropractic Recognition: Prosecution and Legislation in Massachusetts," *Chiropractic History* 2 (1982): 55–65; "Brief Guide for Chiropractic Oral History Research," *Chiropractic History* 5 (1985): 39–40; "Before the Palmers: An Overview of Chiropractic's Antecedents," *Chiropractic History* 7 (December 1987): 27–33; "Chiropractors: Evolution to Acceptance," in *Other Healers*, 157–91.

In 1981, the newly formed Association for the History of Chiropractic published its first *Archives and Journal*, a collection of nine papers presented at its first annual conference on chiropractic history, June 5–6, at the Smithsonian's National Museum of American History. The *Journal* was expressly created as "a scholarly effort" to document chiropractic history. It is a welcome and valuable addition to the literature on chiropractic, but the quality of the articles is uneven and the effort sometimes falls short of the intent. Of the ninety-three articles that appeared in the *Journal* from volume 1, number 1 (1981) through volume 11, number 2 (1991), sixty-one were either written or co-written by Doctors of Chiropractic (D.C.s) or D.C. students. A number of the other articles were written by individuals employed in various capacities by chiropractic colleges. Although this, of course, does not *ipso facto* preclude objectivity, the tone of many pieces indicates the difficulty of maintaining an independent perspective from within the profession.

Medical sociologists as well as historians have been remiss in considering chiropractic as an important social and medical phenomenon, perhaps because of a tendency to assume the viewpoint of the orthodox medical profession. In "Medical Sociology and Chiropractic" (*Sociological Symposium* [Spring 1978]: 1–3), James K. Skipper provided a brief historiography of medical sociology on chiropractic. It is brief for a reason. As Skipper explained, "if all the pages in the medical sociology texts cited above [in his article] were added together, they would equal no more than a short chapter." This issue of *Sociological Symposium* was devoted to "The Sociology of Chiropractors and Chiropractic"; six articles on chiropractic appeared, a beginning attempt to redress this imbalance. Since then Merrijoy Kelner, Oswald Hall, and Ian Coulter produced a sociological study of chiropractic in Canada entitled *Chiropractors: Do They Help?* (Toronto: Fitzhenry & Whiteside, 1980). In "Chiropractic Observed: Thirty Years of Changing Sociological Perspectives," *Chiropractic History* 3 (1983), Ian Coulter noted that, although chiropractors have failed to receive extensive study from sociologists,

> where they have been studied the work has often ignored the most fundamental fact about chiropractic, (that [it] is a system of health care) in favor of its more esoteric features such as its marginality, its cultism, its professionalism, (or lack of it), and its deviant theory of disease. For the most part, these studies have been theses, or based on theses, and more concerned with limited sociological problems than with giving a good descriptive account of chiropractic (p. 43).

Because of its conspicuous presence within the current health system, chiropractic clearly merits serious, nonpartisan examination from a many-sided perspective that moves beyond both limited problems and mere description. *Chiropractic in America* has been an attempt in this direction.

Index

Page numbers in *italics* denote illustrations.